HOMEOPATHY OF THE ABSURD

I

E. M. BEEKMAN

HOMEOPATHY OF THE ABSURD

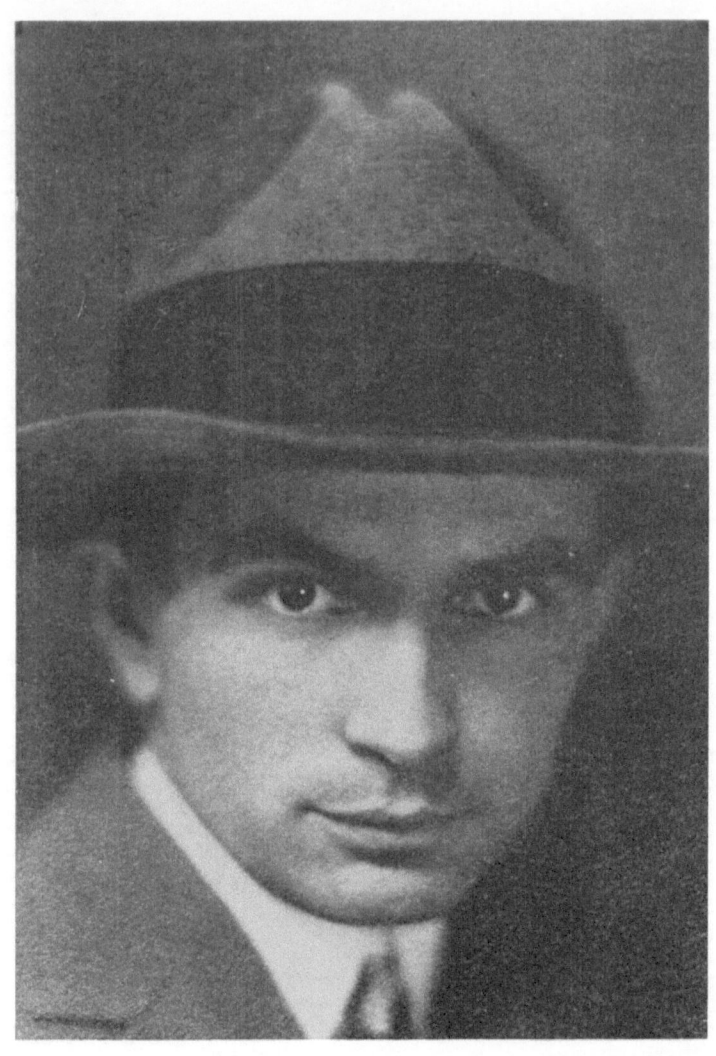

Paul van Ostayen, 1896 - 1928

HOMEOPATHY OF THE ABSURD

The Grotesque in Paul van Ostaijen's Creative Prose

by

E. M. BEEKMAN

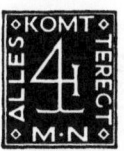

SPRINGER-SCIENCE+BUSINESS MEDIA, B.V.

ISBN 978-94-017-0038-2   ISBN 978-94-015-7580-5 (eBook)
DOI 10.1007/978-94-015-7580-5

TABLE OF CONTENTS

FOREWORD

In many ways a "first," the present study would not be in print without the gracious aid of a number of individuals from both sides of the Atlantic. In the U.S., where this volume constitutes a venture into a literary *terra incognita*, I am indebted to the unflagging support and encouragement of a true gentleman and eminent scholar, Professor Harry Levin. His understanding and humanity will always remain a priceless memory. Professors Henry Hatfield, J. Craig La Drière and Seymour Flaxman were generous with their time and invaluable advice.

The Low Countries were very good to me. Despite his demanding schedule, Prof. Dr. Walter Thys did more than one could normally expect – even from a friend. With such a tireless champion, the international reputation of Dutch Literature should grow with leaps and bounds. The loss of Prof. Dr. Herman Uyttersprot is a grievous one, personally as well as for the profession. To have gained the acquaintance of the great poet Maurice Gilliams is nothing less than an honor. Conversing with him was a liberal education.

Doing research in Belgium as a Fulbright Fellow for 1965–1966 under the auspices of the United States Educational Foundation in Belgium, was made so much easier by Professor Antoine van Elslander and the staff of *Het Seminarie voor Nederlandse Literatuurstudie* at the University of Ghent and Drs. L. Simons, Director of Antwerp's *Archief en Museum voor het Vlaamse Cultuurleven*. The Flemish writer Paul de Vree was, and still is, of great help and remains loyal to Van Ostaijen's cause and his heritage. I am grateful to Drs. Gerrit Borgers, the well-known Van Ostaijen expert, who has been most courteous and generous to me in my efforts to make Van Ostaijen, if not known, at least appreciated by a selected few in the United States. Hence it is a pleasure to acknowledge the existence of some enlightened editors of American periodicals where a number of the translations in the Appendix appeared before in different form: *Mundus Artium*, *The Massachusetts Review*, *New Directions Anthology 21* and *The Chicago Review*.

It is not an easy task to see a work of this nature through the press when the author is some 3000 miles away. Dr. H. J. H. Hartgerink, Director of the Martinus Nijhoff Publishing Company, can only be commended for his patience, expertise and cooperation in making the whole process a pleasant experience.

The man to whom this work is dedicated deserves more than this small token of my love for him. May it be an indication that his wisdom during those difficult years has been justified. My love for Sir Google is gathering interest over the years and only I can gauge the debt I owe Aïda Salomé, que para mi es "el silencio impone su limpidez concreta."

A LABYRINTH FOR OUR TIMES

The redoubtable Sherlock Holmes shows his amazing perspicacity even in such matters as the connotation of words. While Dr. Watson echoes the common interpretation of *grotesque* as "strange-remarkable," Holmes insists that there "is surely something more than that . . . some underlying suggestion of the tragic and the terrible." In adjectival uses *grotesque* usually follows Dr. Watson's explication. The present study elaborates on Holmes' premonition, and is primarily interested in the English phrase *the grotesque* as a concept and a literary genre. It is a term particularly appropriate to a modern mode of fiction, as exemplified in the tales of the Flemish writer Paul van Ostaijen (1896–1928). Current usage retains the popular connotations of several centuries: *grotesque* is a synonym for "strange," "bizarre," for anything distorted or not normal. Such vague usage has made it rather difficult to formulate a precise definition of the grotesque as a literary genre and obscured the original association of carefully contrived unnaturalness, and of the exploration of the darker aspects of fantasy and the imagination.

Most writers on the grotesque agree that the word originated in the sixteenth century as an Italian term to describe peculiar murals which combined vegetal, human and animal forms *ad arbitrium*. The word was applied to this type of art since it was first found, as far as is known, in the chambers or vaults (*grotte*) of Roman buildings, particularly the *Domus Aurea* of Nero excavated in the early sixteenth century. The German scholar G. R. Hocke, in his studies of sixteenth and seventeenth century *Manierismus* (a rich mine for students of the grotesque), designates these murals as "classical grotesques" and traces their origin to ancient grotto-cults.[1] As a literary symbol the grotto, according to Gaston Bachelard, may be related to either "grottes d'effroi" or "grottes d'émerveillement." Even in its origins as word, concept or genre, the grotesque seems to shun any common norms of reality. Edgar Allen Poe, the author of *Tales of the Grotesque and Arabesque*, stressed the grotesque's accent on abnormality in his formula: ". . . the ludicrous heightened into the grotesque, the fearful colored into the horrible, the witty exaggerated into the burlesque, the singular wrought out into the strange and mystical."

The history of *the grotesque* as a concept is surprisingly rich considering the fact that, generally speaking, serious consideration of the term did not start until the eighteenth and nineteenth centuries. The diffuse and elusive connotations of the word itself have produced obstacles for a uniform definition which have still not been surmounted. The grotesque is often associated with the Romantic movement, no doubt because Victor Hugo's manifesto, *Préface de Cromwell* (1827), heralded it as a "type nouveau," though he neglected to specify its characteristics. Hugo is perhaps the most venerable spokesman who started the trend designating the grotesque vaguely as "moyen de contraste," the negative opposite of the sublime. In England, for example, Edmund Burke and Hogarth subscribed to his definition by antithesis. This interpretation is perhaps the most traditional and seems to be the basis, when auxiliary elaborations are ignored, for most of nineteenth century literature on the grotesque, persisting into the first decades of the twentieth century.

According to Arthur Clayborough, who devoted a book to the study of *The Grotesque in English Literature*, Sir Walter Scott was the first to give serious consideration to the grotesque as a genre in English literature. Scott, however, was unwilling to accept the grotesque on its own terms, but would only consider it a beneficial form of writing if it had moral purpose and was aligned to a "traditional atmosphere."[2] Perhaps the major difference between the "traditional" and the "modern" grotesque is the latter's closed world which denies any connection with a naturalistic, moralistic or traditional sphere of reference. The grotesque world of fiction has no need to employ supernatural machinery; it *is* a formulation of an absurd world. "Es ist einfach auf einmal da."[3]

John Ruskin, in *The Stones of Venice*, wrote perhaps the most detailed discourse on the grotesque during the nineteenth century. Ruskin's main ingredients for the "noble grotesque" are horror and beauty, which had become standard fare for the genre during the nineteenth century. But his most interesting contribution to the discussion is his emphasis on the element of play in the grotesque. *Modern Painters* rephrases Ruskin's lengthy argumentation in a succinct summary. The grotesque is "art arising from healthful but irrational play of the imagination in times of rest."[4] For a consideration of the *modern grotesque* the *ludic* element is an important feature.

Clayborough further examines the statements on the grotesque by several other English writers. Walter Bagehot joins hostile critics of the genre by denouncing it as a form of writing which deliberately revels in the ugly and unpleasing aspects of life. Thomas Wright and J. A. Symonds introduce the notion of comic exaggeration into the definition of the term, particularly in the guise of caricature. The importance of this concept as one of the techniques of the grotesque related to its character as a paradoxical form of art has been supported by more modern practioners. Ionesco sees his dramatic technique as "exagération qui disloque le réel," while Dürrenmatt praises the British caricaturist Ronald Searle for his art as "eine der Waffen des menschlichen Geistes, . . . wo die Groteske unversehens zu einer dämonischen Kritik [wird]." [5] The genteel appreciation of the grotesque by George Santayana, when interpreted slightly differently, points to a major requisite of the modern grotesque. His viewpoint is that familiarity with the grotesque does not breed contempt, but ultimately induces a neutralizing effect which renders the grotesque conventional.[6] However, the contention of this study is that this very familiarity with the grotesque universe is a fearful experience. The modern grotesque does not, after a process of familiarization, relapse into conventionality of a quotidian variety, but has come to seem the *only* reality of an absurd universe.

Despite the objections of some critics, Wolfgang Kayser's *Das Groteske in Malerei und Dichtung* still remains a central work for any discussion of the grotesque as a literary genre.[7] Kayser's examination traces the grotesque in German literature from the early eighteenth century up to Kafka. It includes the Romantic movement (especially Friedrich Schlegel, Wackenroder, Tieck, Jean Paul, Hoffman, Kleist), such post-Romantic writers as Keller, Vischer, Busch, and in the present century Wedekind, Schnitzler, Meyrink, Kafka, Morgenstern and Thomas Mann. German literature seems particularly rich in writers as well as critics of the grotesque. One should also include, as will become clear later on, writers of the Expressionistic movement and such contemporary authors as Friedrich Dürrenmatt, Max Frisch and Günther Grass. In his discussion of various authors and aestheticians, and especially in his concluding chapter, Kayser establishes a number of salient characteristics applicable to the modern grotesque and the present study.

i. The grotesque is a fictional structure. This statement might provide an argument against critics who conceive of the grotesque as ramblings dictated by an eccentric fantasy with little control or technical expertise.

ii. The grotesque's fictional structure is that of an alienated world (*entfremdete Welt*). In an attempt to clarify the term "alienated" Kayser pinpoints an important feature, often ignored by critics, of the grotesque. What is alienated is the reader's everyday reality. The grotesque exhibits features readily recognizable, but proceeds to distort these familiar aspects of daily life beyond recognition, into the realm of the absurd. "Es ist unsere Welt, die sich verwandelt hat." This is an important point. The grotesque does not construct a completely invented world of fantasy, but attains its frightening, its uncanny impact from a basis in what is daily reality to us, but which refuses to remain identical to what one conceives to be normal. "Das Grauen überfällt uns so stark, weil es eben unsere Welt ist, deren Verläszlichkeit sich als Schein erweist."

iii. What constitutes the force that induces this alienation remains a critical quandary. Kayser finally settles on a term which has drawn more critical fire than any other element in his book. This absurd force he chooses to call *das Es*, and he does not define it any further. Kayser justifies this antithetically but saying that as soon as "wir die Mächte benennen und ihnen eine Stelle in der kosmischen Ordnung anweisen könnten, verlöre das Groteske an seinem Wesen." Van Ostaijen has a more precise, though practically untranslatable, term for this absurd force. He calls it *verkeerdheid*, which implies a consistently antithetical force as the basis for an entire universe. This term will be discussed below.

iv. "Im Grotesken geht es . . . primär um das Versagen schon der physischen Weltorientierung." Despite the foundation reminiscent of daily reality, the grotesque sets out to destroy normal order. One's accustomed orientation is consistently undermined. The grotesque character has no way out. The unity of perspective in this alienated world is the perspective of the grotesque figures: "in dem kalten Blick auf das Erdentreiben als ein leeres, sinnloses Puppenspiel, ein fratzenhaftes Marionettentheater."

v. When Kayser discusses the problem of humor in the grotesque he mentions an important aspect: the paradoxical element of play. There is definitely an element of the comic in the grotesque but not for enjoyment; it is a grim and ruthless game: "die Gestaltungen des Grotesken sind ein Spiel mit Absurden."

These five major features of Kayser's theory are applicable to Van Ostaijen's grotesques, and will be encountered again in subsequent discussion. One other subdivision of his definition is contestable, however, in terms of the *modern grotesque*. Kayser feels that the act of realizing the negative force in the universe (*das Grauen, das Dunkle*) in art and literature has a liberating function, in that the very act of expression has at the same time the effect of exorcising negativity: "die Gestaltung des Grotesken ist der Versuch, das Dämonische in der Welt zu bannen und zu beschwören." A study of modern forms of the grotesque will reveal that this is not true in most instances. The modern grotesque does not relinquish its inexorable force of the absurd. Generally speaking, the grotesque universe in fiction is ruthless and dictatorial, and gives neither quarter nor solace. In many cases one may speak of a hermetic universe of unconditional folly. Man's natural *horror vacui* is not relieved.

Having very briefly sketched a possible "tradition" of the grotesque in English and German literature, one must consider for a moment the emergence of the grotesque as a major force in modern literature. Naturally, other literatures also have their representatives of the grotesque. In France the work of Rabelais is perhaps the most significant. One may point to elements of the grotesque in Balzac and in the work of authors who wrote *contes fantastiques*, particularly Charles Nodier, Prosper Mérimée and Maupassant. But even more relevant creations of the grotesque in French can be found in the present theatre of the absurd of Ionesco and Beckett. Pirandello, according to Kayser, is representative in this genre of modern Italian literature. Modern Spanish literature has Jorge Luis Borges as its most significant writer of the grotesque, while Russian literature has its past-master in Gogol, examples in Dostoevsky and even such Soviet writers as Zamiatin, Ilf and Petrov, and in Siniavskii, who wrote under the pseudonym of Abram Tertz. But German remains, generally speaking, especially rich in works of the grotesque, and its modern development of the genre is especially significant for a discussion of Van Ostaijen's tales.

Though most contemporary writers do not specify their work as grotesque, many works of fiction of the first half of this century can easily be classified under this heading. In this short introduction one can only hope to approximate a definition of what appears to constitute a genre of the modern grotesque. While most critics still concern themselves largely with eighteenth and nineteenth century manifestations, some admit, though almost in passing, that the period of the past fifty years has been strangely favorable to this type of fiction. Wolfgang Kayser speaks of three periods in German literature when the grotesque was particularly prominent: first, during the sixteenth century, secondly, between the *Sturm und Drang* period and the Romantic period, and thirdly, in modern literature. All three periods share a distrust of previously established order. Such a distrust is not necessarily revolutionary, but can take form in a fictional reflection of a pessimistic scepticism of a current faith in varieties of rationalism. In short, an epochal crisis produces a literary climate in which the grotesque flourishes.

L. B. Jennings, in his study of the grotesque in the Post-Romantic Period in German literature, advances a tempered definition. "The grotesque presents the terrible in harmless disguise, and its playfulness is constantly on the verge of collapsing and giving way to the concealed horror." With a more or less traditional desire for equilibrium, Jennings sees the grotesque as "the balance between the fearsome and the ludicrous aspects." He proceeds to test his thesis on the works of Heine, Immerman, Ludwig, Stifter, Mörike, Keller and Storm – all authors belonging to the period known as Poetic Realism. It is a rather curious choice, since one would find the grotesque only in dormant or recessive form, as Jennings himself admits, for it is a period "where there are few predominantly grotesque works but there is a strong element of subsidiary grotesqueness." Towards the end of his study he touches upon the modern period of German litera-ture, in particular Expressionism, when the modern grotesque came into its own.

This period of Expressionism is also characterized by an extreme prominence of the grotesque itself –naturally, the pessimistically oriented grotesque that ex-presses the terror and ludicrousness of all life. Many collections of so-called *Grotesken* in this period (e.g., those of Meyrink, Ewers, and Scheerbart); and, although the term "Groteske" is a loose one, these works do contain a great deal of the type of grotesque material under discussion. Here the cycle has been com-pleted. *The grotesque is no longer a residue of disorder in an ordered system; it is the immediate reflection of a disordered world. The playful grotesque that restores the comfort of the mind has expanded into the near-tragic grotesqueness of life itself.*[8]

German Expressionism and Dada, which fostered a resurgence of the grotesque, were flourishing during the time when Van Ostaijen was living in Berlin. There he made the acquaintance of at least one writer of the grotesque and read the works of scores of others.

Karl Otten, a former Expressionist, in introducing a collection of Ex-pressionistic grotesques, describes them in terms similar to the five major points of Kayser's definition, the practice of Van Ostaijen and, curiously enough, to certain aspects of *Manierismus* in the late sixteenth and seven-teenth centuries. Otten also sees the grotesque as the result of an epochal crisis, as a "Protest gegen die Zeit und das zeitgenössische Denken..." Like Kayser, Otten states that "das Groteske soll also im Leser oder Be-trachter gewisse schlummernde Wesenszuge seiner Existenz wecken..."[9] The reader is forced out of his normal existence into a world of irreality, having been enticed by an initial similarity which led him into the trap. Kayser concurs: "Der Leser soll aus der Sicherheit seines Weltbildes und aus seiner Geborgenheit inmitten der Tradition und der menschlichen Ge-meinsamkeit herausgerissen werden." Using such terms as *Widerspruch, Gegensatz, Spaltung, Zerrissenheit, Dilemma, Paradoxien, Doppelsinn* and *schizoide Zwangsideen*, Otten makes it clear that incommensurability is the kernel of the grotesque. An antipodal art, the grotesque thrives on deformation. But it is the grotesque's uncanny power to present chaos with the aid of causality. "Immer jedoch gibt sich das krass Alogische, der offenbare Widerspruch zur Erscheinung, den Anschein des alleinig Echten, so dicht umgibt der Dichter mit Kausalität, Natur, Substanz." The writers of the grotesque mock logic, scientific precision and philosophy itself each with its own separate vocabulary, because they "verdrehen Worte so lange, bis niemand mehr weiss, wovon eigentlich die Rede ist." [10]

Otten also emphasizes the fact that most writers of the grotesque are citizens of the modern metropolis. Berlin, where Van Ostaijen lived from 1918 to 1921, was the center of the Expressionistic and the German Dadaistic writers. As "Groszstadt-Dichter," bound to the "Unnatur der Stein- und Betonwüsten," these writers spelled the death of "Naturlyrik, des Natürlichen und damit des Naturalismus." In a letter from Berlin (April 1919), Van Ostaijen writes: "The natural world doesn't interest me so much any more, not even in an activistic sense." [11] This remains true of more contemporary writers of the grotesque. Nevertheless, sometimes a barely perceptible nostalgia can be discerned behind the grim mask of the grotesque. Creators of a ruthless universe, the writers of the grotesque do sense an essential discord between an absurd reality and what, even remotely, might have been possible. But any temptation to sentimentality is crushed by an exaggeration of both the ugly and the beautiful, particularly the ugly. "Das Hässliche wurde in seiner oft grandiösen Schönheit entdeckt und ersetzte im weitesten Umfange das tausendmal als schön gepriesene griechische Idealbild sowohl des Menschen wie der Natur." [12] Finally, the grotesque often expresses itself with *ludic* techniques in order to create a "Sinngebung des Sinnlosen," or as Hocke phrases it: „Wir möchten die Groteske als Ausdruck einer Desintegration bezeichnen." The paradox of using man's *facultas ludendi* to depict a fearful universe stems from the inability to write a tragedy about a world where the absurd is a daily headline. But comedy creates distance, which enables the writer to defy the horrible reality of his world by playing with it.

The art of the grotesque creates its own peculiar style, which consists of "ungewöhnlichen Bildern, Metaphern, Paradoxien, Wortmischungen und Sinnamalgamen." There is an identification of "Wort und Inhalt" as well as "eine innere Schaukelbewegung, die sich von einem Extrem ins andere werfen lässt." [13] Kayser describes a grotesque style as follows: "Was an dieser Rede grotesk wirkt, das ist . . . die Art des Redens, dieses sich überstürzende, Nahes und Fernstes vermischende, alle logische Verknüpfung und jeden festen Satzbau schliesslich sprengenden Reden, das somit als sich vollziehendes und nicht mehr vom Menschenverstand beherrschtes Geschehen sinnfällig wird." The paradoxical style of the grotesque, to be logically illogical, "Nahes und Fernstes vermischende," cannot be achieved by a discourse controlled by the principle of similarity, but rather by a contiguity of disparate elements. Hence, the ideal style of the grotesque work of fiction appears to be one corresponding to Roman Jakobson's formulation of metonymic art.[14] The far-reaching implications of this theory have as yet not been fully explored. For one thing, this theory would provide a critical framework for much of modern prose *and* poetry, though Jakobson restricts his investigation to prose style only. The astonishing parallel between Van Ostaijen's theory and practice and Jakobson's ideas is discussed in some detail in the final section of this study. If only a single instance, it argues for the need of a much wider investigation in modern and contemporary Western literature, as well as for the Flemish writer's incontestable importance and baffling prescience.

As Albert Soergel remarked in an earlier edition of his handbook on Modern German literature: "Für die expressionistische Form ... ist die Groteske nicht mehr ein seltener Grenzfall, sondern eine Lieblingsform der Zeit, zu der alle verneinende Kräfte ebenso hindrängen, wie alle bejahende etwa zur Hymne."[15] Most of the Expressionists wrote something grotesque at one time or another, but Soergel singles out four particular precursors and two "true" writers of the grotesque. A very brief survey of these six authors will sketch the literary backdrop of Berlin around 1920, when Van Ostaijen resided there.

Paul Scheerbart (1863–1915) is the most interesting of these precursors. His works testify to a boundless fantasy, at times apocalyptic. For example, Scheerbart described an imaginary air force at a time when the Wright brothers were developing their first flying machines. He was possessed by cosmic space and his favorite settings for tales often of great lyric beauty were astral bodies, planets, and stars. Van Ostaijen, an avid reader of Scheerbart's work, was attracted by his inventive imagination and "humanity."[16] Soergel describes Scheerbart's works as "grotesken Romanphantasien," wherein he creates "Weltwesen," and dreams of "Geistern, Riesen, Stern- und Weltseelen" according to one of the previously mentioned principles of the grotesque: "Irdisches gibt die Einzelheiten der Beschreibung her, aber alles ist ins Unermessliche gesteigert." It is interesting to note, in view of Van Ostaijen's later stylistic development, that Scheerbart's style seems very much a metonymic one.

Hostile to modern technical developments, Gustav Meyrink (1868–

1932) looked for refuge in occult sciences and strange legends. He achieved fame with his novel *Der Golem* (1915), which is set in the Jewish quarter of Prague and has an artificially created monster for its hero. In this novel and in series of stories, Meyrink shows a marked predilection for *das Grausame*: "Da wird ein Stück Wirklichkeit, das scheinbar nur so, wie die Sinne es aufnehmen, geschildert zu einem Stück kalten Grauens..."[17] Kayser also recognizes this principle of the grotesque in Meyrink's work. "Im 'Golem' aber und in den Erzählungen wird das Dunkel hinter der vordergründigen Welt nicht gedeutet und nicht aufgehellt. Das Groteske entfaltet sich in seinem vollen Wesen."

The major point of interest in the work of Hanns Heinz Ewers (1871–1943) is his denigration of content; form and style must replace the modern "Stoffmangel." In Ewers one finds an early example of using logic to reason a discourse into absurdity. "Mit logischen Beweisen oder mit Bilderfülle eines für möglich hingenommen Erlebnisses suchte Ewers mit Glück die Vorstellung zu erwecken, dass man 'wie ein Blinder in einer höchst wunderbaren Schreckenswelt lebe,' 'von deren Existenz' man 'bisher keine Ahnung hatte.'"[18]

But it was the poet Christian Morgenstern (1871–1914) who proceeded to dislodge language from its accustomed pedestal, twisted it, turned it inside out, made it play a grotesque game with traditional meaning and syntax. Morgenstern taught the writers of the grotesque how to play with language until absurdity has displaced normality. As most critics agree, Morgenstern saw art as the supreme exercise of a *facultas ludendi*. The other major parallel with the theory of the grotesque is Morgenstern's desire "das naive Vertrauen in die Sprache und das von ihr getragene Weltbild [zu] erschüttern."[19]

These four precursors gave the example for the Expressionistic grotesque. Soergel indicates that the writers of this movement added a strong cerebral element (already evident in Morgenstern) to the composition of grotesque art.

Es ist kein Zufall, dass der bezeichnendste Schöpfer grotesker Geschichten ein Philosoph ist, der über Kant, Schopenhauer, Nietzsche, Robert Mayer, aber auch über Jean Paul als Denker und über Georg Grosz geschrieben, Bücher über "Psychologie" und "Logik" und über "Schöpferische Indifferenz" verfasst und einen "Katechismus der Magie, nach Kant und E. Marcus" und einen "Katechismus der Aesthetik, nach Kant" angekündigt hat: Salomon Friedländer (geb. 1871 in Gollantsch in Polen), der sich als Dichter mit der Umkehr des Wortes anonym Mynona nennt.

Mynona (who died in 1946) never relinquished the intellectuality of his

work and attacked many issues of his time with a sophisticated and ruthless-
ly subtle logic. He felt, for instance, that the Freudian universe, centered
around sex, was a naive interpretation of life, and mocked it in a series of
stories; technology he reinterpreted to suit his own peculiar "Feinmechanik"
of the human body. From Mynona, whom he knew personally, Van Ostaijen learned to appreciate cerebral style and acid wit, but he would not
follow the German writer into the latter's optimistic cosmosophy.[20].

Besides Mynona, Soergel classifies Kafka (1883–1924) as the other
"true" writer of the Expressionistic grotesque. This is not the place to
embark on a lengthy discussion of Kafka's art, especially since a formidable
literature on Kafka is available and steadily growing. Suffice it to mention
a few general features which tend to support the contention that Kafka can
also be seen as a writer of the grotesque. Kayser points to the closed world
in Kafka's work as a grotesque principle. It is a world of "geschlossenen
Räumlichkeit, die mit technischen Mitteln erbaute Räumlichkeit," which
is both of this world and *verfremdet*. But Kayser sees Kafka's work as
"latente Grotesken" because he feels that an initial agreement with our
sphere of reference is virtually non-existent, that one enters immediately
an entirely different world. Kafka's world does not have "eigentliche Ver-
fremdungen, weil die Welt von Beginn an fremd ist." But despite the fact
that Kayser speaks of Kafka as an entirely separate genre all by himself,
one would think, in view of recent developments in literature, that Kafka is
very much within the grotesque tradition. He simply forced the possibilities
of the grotesque to their ultimate extreme of paradoxical absurdity. When
Kayser sees in Kafka's world an "Abbau der Welt," a fictional environment
where "dat Sprechen ist der Sprache werdende Abbau selber," one should
be able to see the link to Morgenstern as well as to much fiction that is
being written today. More attention has been given to the German writers
of the grotesque, since they form the tradition in which Van Ostaijen's
tales find their place. Recent epistolary evidence strongly supports this
contention, and has minimized suggestions that Van Ostaijen's peculiar
tales had either English or French precursors.

Paul van Ostaijen lived in Berlin from the fall of 1918 to the fall of
1921, precisely those years when the German capital was a veritable
madhouse. Political revolutions were rocking the foundations of social and
political order. Blood flowed in the streets; the German Navy fought
against Imperial troops, while Karl Liebknecht and Rosa Luxemburg were
openly murdered by the police. Economically, the entire nation was bank-
rupt, and the effect must have been particularly oppressive in the big cities.
Art was also undergoing cataclysmic changes. The first generation of Ex-

pressionists, with their Werfel-like humanitarianism, was either killed during the First World War, or had become largely disillusioned. Dada started its own revolution in Berlin in 1918, a revolution which was not confined to desks, but was defiantly active in the streets and in the denunciation of the political establishment. The only constant factor in Berlin at the time seems to have been anarchy in a bewildering series of disguises. For a young iconoclast like Van Ostaijen, who had just experienced the onset of his own disillusionment, Berlin was an experience which could either destroy him or completely change his perspectives.

He had been a youth during the German occupation of Belgium during the war (he was twenty-two when it ended), and had strong emotional and political sentiments for the unpopular cause of Flemish nationalism. Before he left, Van Ostaijen had already obtained a measure of renown as an *avant-gardist*, not only in personal appearance, but also in print. The Flemish poet Maurice Gilliams, drew this portrait of the artist as a young dandy. "In the evening, on the Keyserlei [the main boulevard in Antwerp to *flàner*], I encountered Orpheus in Biedermeier costume. People stared at him because of his eccentric tie, his red velvet vest and his strange black clothes. Sometimes he wore a pearlgrey macfarlane, and when the wind played with the shoulder flaps, he seemed to have wings like an imperial eagle. In winter one saw him with a cap of otter fur. He had a high, stiff collar on. He was the dandy, the lord in hard, grim Antwerp." (*Vita Brevis*, III, p. 16) At sixteen he had begun to publish articles about the new movements in European art, and urged his generation to follow his example. A high school dropout at seventeen, he published his first volume of poems when he was twenty – a volume which, despite foreign influences, struck a new and important note in modern Flemish poetry. In October of 1918 there appeared his second volume of verse, *The Signal* (*Het Sienjaal*), which had some outspoken political verses, as well as a youthful faith in the creation of a brave new world out of the ashes of the Great War. Written under the overwhelming influence of the original German Expressionistic movement, with its strongly humanitarian inclinations, the volume's naive shrillness and revolutionary fervor seems to have alarmed the authorities, who already had an eye on Van Ostaijen for political demonstrations and participation in anti-government groups and periodicals. Whether his fear of imprisonment was justified or not, Van Ostaijen fled Antwerp and went to Berlin.

Though living under precarious circumstances in a large city rife with political, economical, social and artistic upheavals, Van Ostaijen nevertheless had the opportunity to meet various Expressionistic, Dadaistic and

Futuristic artists and writers. These years in Berlin were the most decisive years in his career and were amazingly productive, considering the circumstances. His flirtation with humanitarianism was completely over. These were the years of agonizing outbursts of revenge and despair revealed in the posthumously published volume of explosive verse *The Banquets of Fear and Pain* (*Feesten van Angst en Pijn,* written 1918–1921) as well as in *Occupied City* (*Bezette Stad,* published in 1921), a most remarkable and technically amazing book of poems about the siege of Antwerp during the First World War. From the few available letters of these years it has become clear that Van Ostaijen became friendly with Mynona, read a great deal of Paul Scheerbart's work and began writing his own grotesques. He seems also to have become personally acquainted with Grosz, Klee, Feininger, Kandinsky, Mehring (a leader of the Dadaists), Rubiner, Schickele and, among many others, Herwarth Walden, the influential leader and publisher of the *Sturm*. Van Ostaijen performed the mammoth task of absorbing the literary and artistic, as well as intellectual developments current at the time. Essays, letters and testimonials from critics show how he became thoroughly familiar with the theory and poetry of Däubler and Stramm, the work of Mondriaan, Picasso, Klee, and a score of Dadaists and Expressionists. When he returned to Antwerp in the fall of 1921, Van Ostaijen became, not surprisingly, the leader of a small group of adventurous spirits in the Belgian literary and artistic worlds, while the majority limped a decade or so behind.

Back in Belgium, Van Ostaijen's life did not become any easier. Though acknowledged by a small group, he was generally regarded suspiciously as an *enfant terrible*. In the remaining seven years of his life he refined his poetry to the lyrical alchemy of his projected, but never published, volume of poems, *The First Book of Schmoll* (*Het Eerste Boek van Schmoll*), continued to write his grotesques, and in a series of essays attempted to educate a hostile audience in the mysteries of modern art. In 1925 he even established an art gallery, where he displayed the works of modern artists. The venture was a failure. During the fall of 1925 it finally became obvious that Van Ostaijen was suffering from tuberculosis. Trying to conquer the disease, he began a short odyssey of small, private sanatoria, which ended with his death in March 1928 in Miavoye-Anthée, a tiny hamlet in the Belgian Ardennes.

Paul van Ostaijen is an astonishing phenomenon in literature. Grudgingly condoned by the literary Establishment in his own country while he was alive, writing in a language few people know and the majority still consider some curious offshoot of German, Van Ostaijen reflects in his work many literary, artistic and intellectual developments which only recently have become legitimate. With a bare minimum of schooling, he became one of the most erudite and advanced artists of his time. His lyricism reflects the stylistic revolutions of Mallarmé, Apollinaire, Stramm, and of the Expressionistic, Dadaistic and Surrealistic movements. As subsequent pages will attempt to describe, his creative prose has perhaps found its true significance in the light of postwar developments in fiction. Parallelisms with phenomenology and Jacobson's theory of metonymic art, which will be discussed in the final section, are startling as well as profound. The renewal of interest in his work in Holland, Belgium and Germany testifies to Van Ostaijen's contemporaneity. The work of Paul van Ostaijen must finally take its place in the forefront of modern Western literature.

The following examination of Van Ostaijen's grotesques, although primarily concerned with a descriptive analysis of the Flemish writer's art, is intended to give a concurrent description of what may be called the *modern* or *contemporary grotesque*. Most critics of this genre generally formulate their views on the basis of material provided them by eighteenth and nineteenth century authors. However, in the fiction produced since the Second World War (particularly during the Fifties and Sixties), a strong resurgence of the grotesque has appeared. In recent American fiction, advocates of "black humor" are, essentially, writing a literature of the modern grotesque. As one "black humorist" puts it in a recent anthology, there is a "very fading line," an "almost invisible line ... between fantasy and reality" in our present society; *The New York Times* is "the source and fountain and bible of black humor."[21] Friedrich Dürrenmatt, the contemporary Swiss advocate of the grotesque, concurs: "Ich bin eigentlich nur dann vom Weltuntergang überzeugt, wenn ich Zeitungen lese." Thomas Mann concludes that the grotesque is "the most genuine style" of modern art. Again it is Dürrenmatt who clearly saw the two positions as illustrative of our modern art: "Unsere Welt hat ebenso zur Groteske geführt wie zur Atombombe, wie ja die apokalyptischen Bilder des Hieronymus Bosch auch grotesk sind." The previously quoted critic Jennings, who subscribes to a more traditional interpretation of the grotesque, must finally admit that, in the present age, the grotesque is not a form of art which makes the demonic trivial, but is "the immediate reflection of a disordered world." One American critic even claims the grotesque as "an American genre."[22] Kayser's statement is more sweeping: "Die Kunst der Gegenwart zeigt eine Affinität zum Grotesken wie vielleicht keine andere Epoche."

Dürrenmatt considers the grotesque a potent force for his own and his contemporaries' art, and explains its relevance to the time in which he is living. "Doch das Groteske is nur ein sinnlicher Ausdruck, ein sinnliches Paradox, die Gestalt nämlich einer Ungestalt, das Gesicht einer gesichtslosen Welt, und genau so wie unser Denken ohne den Begriff des Paradoxen nicht mehr auszukommen scheint, so auch die Kunst, unsere Welt, die nur noch ist, weil die Atombombe existiert: aus Furcht vor ihr." In the modern grotesque, therefore, there is little escape into morality, beauty, the sublime, but there is rather the desperate attempt to render the *essential* absurdity of the world which confronts the author. Van Ostaijen called it the world's basic *verkeerdheid*; Karl Otten a "Sinngebung des Sinnlosen." The modern grotesque is basically pessimistic and, at the same time, a vehement protest against modern times.

To express a cosmic chaos requires the grotesque to employ paradox as a basis for its art: "Im Paradoxen erscheint die Wirklichkeit." [23] One expression of paradox is an alogical loquacity which could reason about the most absurd situations with the best of ancient Sophists. The Polish critic Jan Kott, presenting a modern appreciation of Shakespeare, interprets *King Lear* as a dramatization of the grotesque. "The Fool uses dialectics, paradox and an absurd kind of humor. His language is that of our modern grotesque. The same grotesque that exposes the absurdity of apparent reality and of the absolute by means of a great and universal reductio ad absurdum." G. R. Hocke has a pithy definition for the modern grotesque: "Wahnsinn nach Regeln."

Paradox, as the kernel of grotesque art and style, produces a comic mode which is the laughter of despair, laughter that annihilates – Jean Paul's "vernichtende Idee des Humors." For Dürrenmatt, comedy is the best form of dramatic expression in modern literature. But it is not comedy for relaxation, nor even the comic mode of the bizarre and strange which so often has been designated as the basis for the grotesque. "Die Komödie ist eine Mausefalle, in die das Publikum immer wieder gerät und immer noch geraten ist." The humor of the grotesque does not relieve, but turns deadly serious. "The grotesque is a criticism of the absolute in the name of frail human experience. That is why tragedy brings catharsis, while the grotesque offers no consolation whatsoever." [24] Grotesque humor is a direct reflection of the grotesque's paradoxical nature, of its realization of the bitter irony that fact bypasses fiction: Jean Paul's "klaffende Kontrast zwischen Form und Stoff." "Es ist ein Humor ohne Heiterkeit." [25]

Johan Huizinga's thesis of Western man as *homo ludens* has become the contemporary artist's only serious attitude to his material. [26] But his game is a game with the absurd. It is a game seemingly without rules. But the ostensible freedom of the modern grotesque, which could be seen as a direct

reflection of chaotic madness, is, among its best practioners, a license which
deceives. "Freiheiten beruhen auf Spielregeln, welche die Macht innehält,
um nicht als solche zu scheinen."[27] The implication is a conscious control of
the medium. Indeed, the modern grotesque is a sophisticated and cerebral
mode of fiction. The caricatures of Ronald Searle are an "art" which needs
to be "learned," according to Dürrenmatt, and he adds that "die Satire ist
eine exakte Kunst." About his own work Dürrenmatt, perhaps the most
important apologist for the modern grotesque, says curtly, "ich schreibe
prinzipiell keine Stücke für Dummköpfe." The modern grotesque is therefore
"eine Angelegenheit des Witzes und des scharfen Verstandes"; it consists of
what Wieland called "Hirngeburten."[28] *Alogic* and a rigorous intellectuality
may be polar principles but, as Hugo Friedrich remarks, they go hand in hand
in modern literature.

A calculated mutiny, the modern grotesque creates its own autonomous
universe: "es ist exakte Wiedergabe einer mysteriosen Wirklichkeit."[29] A
ruthless universe created with great precision, the modern grotesque gives
no quarter, nor does it allow escape from its trap. The grotesque does not
permit its inhabitants to transcend their habitat; it does not, as one critic
suggested, affirm "the assertive spirit."[30] "Diese Kunst will nicht mitleiden
wie die Tragödie, sie will darstellen."[31] Such an autonomous and escape-
proof stockade of absurdity and chaos makes the reader hardly entertain
the notion of a symbiosis between author and product. Van Ostaijen is
careful to point out, in his essay on Breughel, how the artist of the grotesque
practises an art of distance; familiarity with the subject breeds contempt.
Dürrenmatt is one of the very few modern commentators to have recognized
this important feature of distance. He manages to combine the two polar
distinctions of the grotesque, its contemporaneity and its distinctive brand
of humor, which thrives in the distance which the author maintains between
himself and his work.

> Es ist nicht zufällig, dass Aristophanes, Rabelais und Swift kraft des Grotesken
> ihre Handlungen *in* ihrer Zeit abspielen liessen, Zeitstücke schrieben, *ihre* Zeit
> meinten. Das Groteske ist eine äusserste Stilisierung, ein plötzliches Bildhaft-
> machen und gerade darum fähig, Zeitfragen, mehr noch, die Gegenwart aufzu-
> nehmen, ohne Tendenz oder Reportage zu sein. Ich könnte mir daher wohl eine
> schauerliche Groteske des Zweiten Weltkrieges denken, aber *noch* nicht eine Tra-
> gödie, da wir noch nicht die Distanz dazu haben können.

The modern grotesque is not a construction of pure absurdity as Karl
Guthke suggests,[32] but as the brief sketch of the history of the grotesque
indicated, it includes the real, daily world as *Stoff.* "Die Fiktion muss auch
die 'wirkliche Welt' in sich enthalten . . . die Fiktion darf nicht als blosse

Absurdität konzipiert werden. Das Absurde umschliesst nichts."[33] Hence
the modern grotesque performs a remarkable feat. The writer creates a
world of the absurd as an impersonal force which makes use of daily
reality as material for its construction, and employs the comic mode to
preserve distance and at the same time to trap his audience in his fictional
world, where it is then forced to listen. A comical "Verrätselung," the
grotesque presents the world as "ein Ungeheures . . . als ein Rätsel an Un-
heil, das hingenommen werden muss, vor dem es jedoch kein Kapitulieren
geben darf."[34]

Combining all the paradoxical features and qualities of the modern grotesque, one may call it a labyrinthean dance. "Es ergibt sich eine Kombi-
nation vom ingeniös-tragischer Verirrung (im labyrinthischen Teil des ver-
wickelten Tanzes) und von Harmonie und von Grotesken. Es vereint also
auch und gerade dieser Tanz das Gegensätzliche in bezeichnender Art und
Weise."[35] The modern grotesque is an ingeniously constructed labyrinth
for our times.

Finally, a brief comment on the similarity between Van Ostaijen and
recent American authors. Leslie Fiedler, though never speaking of the grotesque, characterizes modern American fiction as the "negative novel" in
terms very similar to those just discussed.

The vision of the truly contemporary writer is that of a world not only absurd
but also chaotic and fragmentary. He tries in his work to find techniques for representing a universe in which our perceptions overlap but do not coincide, in which
we share chiefly a sense of loneliness: our alienation from whatever things finally
are, as well as from other men's awareness of those things and of us. Rapid shifts
in point of view; dislocations of syntax and logic; a vividness more like halluci-
nation than photography; the use of parody and slapstick at moments of great
seriousness; the exploitation of puns and of the vaudeville of dreams – these experiments characterize much of the best work of recent decades, from Joyce's
Ulysses through Djuna Barnes' *Nightwood* to Wright Morris' *Field of Vision*,
whose winning of the National Book Award so incensed the guardians of middle-
brow standards.[36]

At the time they were written a relatively singular phenomenon, Van
Ostaijen's grotesques can now be understood in the light of both a "tra-
ditional' development and such a contemporary development as modern
American fiction. For an American audience, it might provide a basis for
comparison to juxtapose the Flemish writer with such current authors as
Joseph Heller, Thomas Pynchon, William S. Burroughs, James Purdy, Kurt
Vonnegut Jr., John Barth and Donald Barthelme. In England comparisons
may be made with Harold Pinter's theatre and screenplays, Samuel Beckett,
Tom Stoppard, and aspects of the work of Anthony Burgess, Iris Murdoch

and Muriel Spark. True to the tradition previously mentioned, there are several important contemporary writers of the grotesque in the German language: Friedrich Dürrenmatt, Günter Grass, Max Frisch and, at times, Heinrich Böll.

One may well ask whether any of these authors who illustrate the theory of entropy in their work have anything left to believe in. When one is preoccupied with a fictional homeopathy of the absurd (*similia similibus curantur*), what constant could possibly survive? Leslie Fiedler provides the correct answer in his previously mentioned work.

In the end, the negativist is no nihilist, for he affirms the void. Having endured a vision of the meaninglessness of existence, he retreats neither into self-pity and aggrieved silence nor into a realm of beautiful lies. He chooses, rather, to render the absurdity which he perceives, to know it and make it known. To know and to render, however, mean to give form; and to give form is to provide the possibility of delight – a delight which does not deny horror but lives at its intolerable heart.

The writers of the Expressionistic grotesques agreed that "Ernst genommen wird nur die Kunst, der dichterische Ausdruck."[37] The final section of this study of Van Ostaijen also indicates his faith in the creative act, in being "simply a poet." Within the context of Dutch and Flemish criticism, the present examination of Van Ostaijen's creative prose simply stresses a unity of style and a unity of vision. For those for whom his work (and that of those modern authors mentioned before) remain a reason for discontent, one can only adjoin Friederich Dürrenmatt's exhortation: "Das Beste an der heutigen Weltanlage ist noch, dass die Schriftstellerei wieder anfängt, gefährlich zu werden."

UNITY OF THEME:
A TOPOGRAPHY OF THE GROTESQUE

The well-known Dutch critic, Garmt Stuiveling, supports a negative opinion of Paul van Ostaijen's prose work. His comments betray perplexity and a reluctance to allow Van Ostaijen's work a permanent place in the development of modern literary history. Van Ostaijen's achievement, especially that of the tales, continues to bewilder even some of the more sophisticated interpreters. Critical mystification expresses itself in terms of barely concealed denigrations: experimentation, inaccessibility, five-finger exercises, diffuse multiplicity.[1] No one would ever assert that Van Ostaijen smoothed a path for the critic; he made no concessions to his readers. But he did not wilfully erect a fence to keep out intruders. A relatively large body of critical commentary on his own and his contemporaries' artistic endeavors indicates his desire to provide a theoretical correlative to his artistic productions. In most cases a patient reading of these theoretical writings would illuminate the alleged opacity of his work. Such an endeavor would refute the contention that the prose work contains inscrutable experiments without unity or pattern. Most tales share a common narrative perspective. Tracing the major ramifications of this fictional world necessitates the exclusion of many details. Their exclusion is a sacrifice to the emphasis on the tales' overall thematic unity.*

PESSIMISTIC BURLESQUES: VAN OSTAIJEN AND BREUGHEL

Among Van Ostaijen's various essays on art and artists, his essay on Breughel constitutes a theoretical draft of the thematic concordance of the tales. The essay is much more than a critical review of Karl Tolnai's book *Die Zeichnungen Pieter Breugels* (München, 1925). Being more than a testimonial of an accidental affinity, the essay reveals Van Ostaijen's reflections on the world of the grotesque. For his own purposes the essay tried to rectify

---

* See the Appendix for a chronology of Van Ostaijen's tales.

stereotyped erroneous interpretations of Breughel's work, while in the context of the present study it clarifies the critical quandary concerning these tales.

The key tone of pessimism is struck in the introductory paragraph. Van Ostaijen insists that Breughel's work does not celebrate Flemish sensuality. On the contrary, a confrontation with Breughel's work should instill in the viewer "the bitter knowledge of the emptiness of human effort."[2] Breughel teaches the "platonic-pessimistic acceptance of futility" and "the hopelessness of action and chaos-creating human restlessness." (IV, 278) These three utterances are slightly modified variations on the central theme of resigned pessimism, which negates the world and human action in a consistent fashion. Van Ostaijen's pessimism is not a artificial pose, but is basic to both his life and work. In a letter from Berlin (April, 1919) he confesses his pessimistic intentions in the grotesques. "Wrote a novella in which I try to make monkeys of people. Positive criticism: baloney. Now I like novellas in which you can fool around so marvelously. People aren't worth criticizing. Only material for burlesque novellas."[3] The tale "Jus primae noctis" may be seen as a condensed record of Van Ostaijen's nihilism. In this story, where fictional elements have been stripped to a bare, somewhat Platonic dialogue, Van Ostaijen's *persona* confesses: "Pessimism in itself as a view of life would be deliverance for me. And a great wealth. This I cannot have. Everything has become flat for me, because I did not desire the abstract consistently. Consider this pessimism with comparisons oriented to the world at large. Everything is such a pitiful mess." (III, 13)

Speaking about his lyricism, Van Ostaijen uses terms similar to those in his discussion of Breughel's work. Van Ostaijen's pessimism – more a tempered nihilism reminiscent of Alfred de Vigny and the Flemish poet Maurice Gilliams – does not however degrade itself into breastbeating, anarchy or destructive rebellion, but simply sees life's futility as a condition and accepts its consequences. Futility and the insuffiency of expression are central to his art. Inability of language ever to catch satisfactorily the most profound pattern which underlies our lives and environment, as well as the futility of man's endeavors, is contained in the following passage from a key-essay on the uses of poetry.

Poetry does not originate only from the daemonic, but also from the shock between the daemonic force of the word and the awareness of the hopelessness of every human attempt at formulation. Between these two: the will to express and the hopelessness of expression there is a constant interaction and perhaps often strife. And the more one gains possession of the means which allow one to catch the daemonic on the surface, the more one begins to doubt the effectiveness, the absolute truth of these means. As far as consciousness can exercise its power, the daemonic ultimately yields to hopelessness and this reality, valid for me, I can already illustrate with the fact that, for me, no poem about the phenomenon "fish" could ever be more powerful than this word *fish* itself. (IV, 316)

One might easily predict, given the symptoms, an artistic impotence, a turning away from life – contemplating the Empedoclean crater's edge. Van Ostaijen, like most modern artists who see their art through a glass darkly, bravely instituted faith in the creative act. They recognize the fact that creation may negate, or at least neutralize, the spectre of depression. For, says Van Ostaijen, "the lyrical emotion is a negation of a pessimistic view of life." (IV, 317)

Other important premises are implied in the essay's first paragraph. An element of frustration, hidden in the diction, indicates a residual aggression which prevents total apathy. Frustration is the kinetic force of his grotesques. With vehement indignation, Van Ostaijen attacks the prevailing notion that Breughel reveled in bawdy and gross sensuality.[4] In his discourse on Breughel's style and vision, which runs counter to the Rabelaisian stereotype, Van Ostaijen delineates his own peculiar view of narrative fiction. The artist is an impartial observer of the world's folly. Van Ostaijen stresses the formality, objectivity and cerebrality of Breughel's art. The artist distances himself from the world he depicts. "And even in his *Peasant Wedding* or in his early *Dutch Proverbs*, does one not see the distance which separates the painter from this world, does one not see with how much objectivity he faces these events, almost as if all this belonged to the goings on of a species alien to him." (IV, 280) The notions of estrangement and alienation which Van Ostaijen implies in the last clause are equally basic to his own narrative fiction. A *Verfremdungseffekt* emanates from the consistent objectivity. A sequential series of related concepts can be derived from the basic divorce between artist and subject. Soon technique and content of Breughel's antithetical art run parallel courses in Van Ostaijen's discussion.

Breughel, according to Van Ostaijen, does not take part in the peasant vulgarity he depicts. Disjunction between the artist and his product follows from a critical scepticism. The act of creation is an extraneous one. No longer is the artist and his subject the creative symbiosis familiar from the Romantic era: "Breughel himself is not at home in his paintings." (IV, 280) Neither rejecting nor accepting, the artist notes in a neutral fashion the object of his interest. The object constitutes the notation; the notations are a stenographic record of a world awry. Van Ostaijen does perceive, but almost begrudgingly, a minimal amount of involvement on the part of

Breughel. "At the most one could say of Breughel that he is amused by the grotesqueness of the object of this notation, but he is not delighted by it as much as Swift amuses himself in the notation of the follies Gulliver gradually discovers in people, nor does he, indeed, even less than Swift who was more apostolic, have any relation to this world of absurdity." (IV, 281) This statement, couched in Van Ostaijen's peculiar yet subtle style and finely nuanced thought, obliquely comments on the curious brand of humor in a tale of the grotesque. Previously he had negatively asserted that one is not amused by the grotesque condition. Now he proceeds to qualify this statement. The nature of the notation may betray a grim amusement on the part of artist, but he cannot be said to disport himself. The latter would obviously constitute involvement and a certain sense of agreement. Such a relationship would be contradictory to the axiomatic negation of the object and its rendition. Van Ostaijen also refutes the contention that there is a moralizing force in Breughel's paintings; he feels that, intrinsically, the grotesque work of art does not moralize. But Van Ostaijen is somewhat dogmatically inclusive here. Surely, if the artist does not include an ethical norm within the autonomous work itself, this does not mean the exclusion of a critical interpretation of the completed body of work. The image on the retina makes no judgment; the mental verdict lies in the focus. Choice betrays involvement.

Van Ostaijen makes exteriorization a central feature of Breughel's art, as he already had made it of his own work. Breughel, he feels, remained objective and at a distance from what he created. Hence the exterior reality he creates is an inevitable result of the medium of painting and the subject, but it does not betray the artist's own personality. The work of art remains master within its own domain. "Le seul aspect mystérieux que présente 'l'extérieur' est une conséquence du fait qu'il n'est pas autre chose qu'extériorisation. Représenter l'extérieur sans l'extériorisation équivaut à la représentation d'une fausse réalité: imprimer des billets de banque sur du papier de journal. Peindre cet extérieur multiplié avec la conscience qu'il n'est pas autre chose qu'extériorisation, c'est peindre vrai et représenter un mystère exact." (IV, 137) In literature as well as painting, Van Ostaijen wants to establish an impersonal art; the gauge for such an art-form is disindividualization. This concept is repeatedly alluded to in the essays. Cubism, as Van Ostaijen charts its course, had advanced artistic expression from a "subjective-revolutionary" period to a modern, superior one of disindividualization. In a manifesto for a periodical which never saw the light but which was to have been the organ for "emancipated Cubism" or "organic Expressionism," the three central preoccupations of Van Ostaijen's theoretical writings are summarized in a few sentences: the work of art as an organism, its autonomous existence, and the disindividualization of the artist. "The work of art is an organism. *The work of art is a living entity.* As such it is *in itself* individual in the primary sense of the word, in itself indivisible. The task, therefore, from the point of view of the artist is: disindividualization." (IV, 84)

Particularly in the case of poetry, this endeavor should result in an anonymity of the work of art, in a true communality of art. Communal art does not necessarily mean an art comprehensible to the masses, but is more a formulation of a striving for disindividualization. Communal art, therefore, stands for a wide application of the desire to set the work of art free, to accept it on its own terms without the interference of the artist's personality. Not the poet, but the poem is important. The immediate analogy which comes to Van Ostaijen's mind is the anonymous literature of nursery rimes, ancient ballads and folk songs. A modern form which would emulate those nameless folk artists should intensify the objectivity of expression and of the artist's personality in such a way that the poem, and the poem alone, will demand attention while its creator remains a nameless artificer; "... one must strive for a poetry which would be the popular lyricism made by poets one step higher, these are poets whose awareness of the esthetic is *a priori* greater than that of the folk poet." (IV, 291)

The style of the grotesques stresses an objectivity of expression. Van Ostaijen remains in most cases an impersonal recorder of a world of absolute folly. The unifying style of the grotesques and their abstract quality only force all the more attention on the subject of an incongruous world. Naturally, in the grotesques the subject is more important than in the poems, and the manner of the exposition forces the reader to continually reevaluate their common denominator of folly; the various manifestations of this essential vision, be it sex, chauvinism or counterfeiting, are merely refractions of this basic theme. The grotesques are the negative expressions of the poetic theory. While Van Ostaijen strove in his poetry for pure lyricism, he attempted to express with similar means (subject to the modifications of prose) an objective configuration of a negative world; i.e., stripped of an author's individual intrusions. As does the poetry, the grotesques establish their own autonomous microcosm by eliminating the author from its independent domain.

An immediate negative response to these theoretical concepts might be the accusation of inertia. In his lyrics, Van Ostaijen wanted to create tension through the printer's blank spaces in various controlled distances between components of a line of verse. The measure of separation was for him the tension between two parts in a lyrical line divided by the white space. Lyrical tension was either assonance or dissonance; dissonance he felt to be self-explanatory, while he described the effect of assonance as either strengthening or neutralizing the preceding element in a line of verse. (IV, 205) The fixity of the prose tales gives them a tension-quotient of their own. Their apparent immobility reveals, at closer examination, an inner dynamism; tension results from combining their architectonic modality of style and their latent chaos. Van Ostaijen describes this phenomenon in a discussion of James Ensor's paintings of masks.

> In his imagination he posits objects which, with the artist's obvious approval, stiffen in the most comical rigidity. Outwardly there is no more pronounced immobility than these stupid masks. All the features are rigid; each mask is a death-mask. But when one looks more closely at the works than in normal comfort, one comes very soon to the conclusion that this stiff outer rigidity has been willed for the strong antagonism with a very carefully thought-out inner dynamism. This antagonism is carried out down to the most insignificant details. (IV, 29)

The point which must be reiterated again and again is that Van Ostaijen insists that what seems to us superficially incommensurate with our traditional notions of enjoyment only appears so because the work of art is not to be experienced according to a set of preconceived individual notions. The work of art is *einfach existent*, in and for itself. Our sphere of reference must be shifted from a personal conglomeration of culturally conditioned reflexes to the organic existence and separate legality of the work of art *an sich*. *Verfremdung*, in this sense, is merely a severance of the artist and his product. The sympathetic umbilical cord has been cut, and the created product lives on its own, a planet in its own galaxy. This is probably the reason for the pedagogic bent of Van Ostaijen's essays. The new movement in art demands a reeducation of its audience in terms of the individual work of art, which has its own laws, proportions, and relationships, and the movement tries to eradicate the usual identification of the artist's existence as expressed in his work. *Einfach existent*. The hermetic, self-sufficient world of the poem, painting, or grotesque has a democracy all its own. The most contradictory forces are relevant within the totality of the creative autocracy.

Van Ostaijen's philosophical speculations about Breughel's art tempts the reader to see parallel profundities in Van Ostaijen's work. But this problematic relevance would be more applicable to his poetry than his prose; noting that the latter's predominant theme is that of a world out of joint, must suffice here. Speculation about Platonic connotations in the tales would needlessly complicate the relative simplicity of their meaning. This is not to deny that the tales invite speculations of this sort. The very incommensurability of the grotesque world invites speculation about the X-factor of the equation – incommensurable with what? Negation prefigures ideality. But the world of the grotesque restricts itself to quintessential otherness – a *de facto* condition. However, certain terms in Van Ostaijen's essay are quite relevant to this discussion. Nature and the world of man are sharply divided in Breughel; one is reason, the other irrationality. Basic incommensurability between man's endeavors and an ideal (in the case of Breughel, primordial nature) is amplified throughout the essay. In terms of the grotesque, it is one of its basic features. A chasm, a sense of nil, permanently separates the grotesque world of consistent otherness from the X of the implied equation. Sympathetic reciprocation is impossible. Rapidly the minus pole of this proposition intensifies its negativity until the ultimate deduction has been made; the grotesque is a world of absolute absurdity.

This is a world of folly enacted by anorganic puppetry. The metaphor imparts inhuman, mechanical features to this chaos. In "Claire's Herd," for example, the relationship between Claire and her following, the *rastas*, is described in terms of a puppeteer and his marionettes. Notice that Van Ostaijen emphasizes the unimportance of the subject of Claire's games with the *rastas*, since the stereotyped participants allow little or no dramatic variation. The *rastas* are set into motion by a mechanical force over which they have no control whatsoever.

Claire was in the same situation with the rastas as the owner of a Punch and Judy show with his actors. She improvised the actual plays as she saw fit, did not stick to a specific text. The puppet-show was open to her, she had only to choose . . . As long as she noticed something alive, something like free will in a puppet, the puppet interested her. But if she had seen through the puppet and understood it as a clock-work – exclusion of free will-hypothesis; every gesture and every sound are forced by the movement of a spring – then it's over. Claire was no different. The gestures and the dialogue – intonation as well as subject – are limited and quasi stereotyped . . . Their nature is such that they must imitate each other; one can't say aping, it is a stronger reflex-action. The typical distinction is similar to that of puppets. Only for a while can one really believe in that typical distinction; one grows tired of one rasta after the other, just as a child of one doll after the other. In this manner Claire played with the rastas. Grabbed one after the other. Discovered suddenly that one was exactly like the other. Threw it back and allowed herself to be enticed by the gestures of a third, which appeared to her at first to be new again. (III, 299–300)

This passage is an accurate description of the characters in these tales, of their uniformity and their mechanical behavior.

Folly is an immanent force which rules life in the world of the grotesque. A *ne plus ultra*, it will not allow such divagations as quotidian normality. It is anonymous, dictatorial, ruthless and inhuman. Van Ostaijen found the perfect metaphor to symbolize these qualities – the modern corporation. Van Ostaijen's world of absolute *verkeerdheid* is Folly Incorporated. Folly, in this context of the grotesques, has no redemptive or extenuating qualities. This is no fatuous folly or levity. *Verkeerdheid* implies want, absence, derangement; in terms of these tales it has a demonic inevitability which corresponds, to some degree, to μαυία from μάυεθαι "to be mad." An element of manical desire for derangement of the norm is couched in a sinister, destructive urge. But one particular aspect must be kept in mind; its anarchy is not chaotic. The very symbol of the organization pledges order. It is a world of perspicacity, structure, authority, argumentation and rationalization, just like the world of our daily lives. The difference lies in the fact that this world is constructed on a foundation of anarchy. Behind the looking glass of reality lies a world reflected from our world, similarities between the two are inversely proportional to our standards. Through the looking glass lies a world gone amok in a logical manner. "Die Welt geht umgekehrt als es richtig wäre! Die Gegenwart ist hinter sich in die Vergangenheit sehend, Geburt liegt hinten, und vorn liegt der Tod. Es ist 'ne böse ganz verdrehte Geschichte. Jemand hat die Kurbel rückwärts gedreht. Und wer trotzdem vorwärts will, der hat es verflucht schwer und richtet wenig aus. Das ist kein Bild, kein Gleichnis, Sie dösiger Affe: sondern die Sache selbst." [5]

Discussing technique and its conceptual implications in Breughel's art, Van Ostaijen provides us with oblique insight into his own intentions. Stylistically, nuances are of great importance. The depiction of Promethea in "Ika Loch's Brothel" is a sum of graphic distinctions. She, like most characters in Van Ostaijen's grotesque world, is from a psychological point of view, virtually non-existent. Their very one-dimensionality lends them a stilted grace and presence despite atrophy of the fictional skeleton. This method of writing has, stylistically, features of the graphic medium of art. Speaking of Breughel's art, Van Ostaijen's fictional techniques assume contour and content. The serried quality of style provides anonymity. Modulation would pierce through uniform matter. Rigidity, however, preserves the grotesque in a state of suspended animation. Van Ostaijen's fictional technique resembles that of the animated cartoon. The precision which goes into granting a one-dimensional figure the illusion of motion is like the hypertrophied stylization of the tales. Yet the cartoonist knows full well that each act of motion is a single drawing of immobile contours and graphite volume. For example, at any point in a series of drawings depicting a character opening its mouth, the development can be halted. A projector stopped at an absurd gesture might thus lend it a peculiar timelessness of expression. An example in which this process was seemingly applied to an entire story is "Ika Loch's Brothel." Having denigrated logic at length with alogical loquacity, the brothel's figures vanish behind a description of the building's interior. The next to the last sentence freezes the roaming eye of the fictional camera on "a nightvase with a deep red rose." Simplicity of the poetic image harbors a vast domain of profound mystery. In its terse poetic mystification, it is categorically antithetical to the preceding verbose rationalization of incongruity. One sentence, a single poetic image, throws an entire verbal structure out of kilter. A frozen metaphor's mysterious presence mocks the grotesque's insidious intent.

The carefully contrived verbal structures of the grotesque cannot hide their fraudulent objective. These intricately built tales are a senseless architecture. The foregoing example from "Ika Loch's Brothel" seems to support this contention. Nevertheless, the grotesque impresses one with its autonomous existence. Within its walls martial law has been declared. Hence it does not allow identification between the reader's sphere of reference and that of the grotesque. They must remain separate; it is not a matter of identification. Yet must remain separate; it is not a matter of identification. Yet the grotesque slyly impresses the reader with a sense of *déjà vu*. A grotesque is not a non-representational painting. Deformation implies a basis of form. A tale of the grotesque will use a familiar concept, instance or trait and proceed to develop it beyond normality. But in order to be effective, it must have some relevance to a normal sphere of reference. For example, patriotic sentiment becomes an international enterprise which regulates war and peace as a matter of business ("Patriotism Incorporated"). The commendable desire for metropolitan beautification turns into a building craze without rhyme or reason ("City of Builders"). In a world where economy equals inflation, counterfeit bills are more honest currency than legal tender ("The Adventures of Mercurius"). The stereotyped slogan "Work and Save" carried to an extreme does not benefit, but victimizes its apostle. Perhaps most graphically illustrative is "The Lost House Key," where a victim of satyriasis loses his house key, and with this insignificant act, becomes the founding father of a syphilitic society. Indeed, a pessimistic vision might conclude that any of these grotesque deformations have their place in our universe. Van Ostaijen sees his world as a panopticon where nothing is unnatural, or, at most, against nature. The world of the grotesque has the disturbing tendency of appearing familiar to us, and yet we desperately insist on its alien character.

The grotesque is a double-edged sword. It terrorizes its actors as well as its audience. This fearful oscillation between repugnant familiarity and alien autocracy was what perplexed the Dutch critic mentioned previously. "As long as we are reading, we have the oppressive feeling that all this bizarre, strange and sometimes grisly business does concern us in a mysterious fashion, because it depicts a piece of a hidden reality in which we take just as much part as the author. It is a spell which does not fascinate us, but renders us helpless, from the inside out. We cannot recount what we experienced; it does not go deeper or higher than cognition, but bypasses it." [6] The irony of this statement must be obvious, since it reflects an impression *intended* by the grotesque. But the grudging admission does not hide repulsion. Correcting the critical focus results in the realization that the diagnosis of the symptoms correctly identified the disease.

THE WORLD OF VAN OSTAIJEN'S GROTESQUES: SYPHILIZATION

The best fictional counterpart to these theoretical statements is the story "The Lost House Key." Counterpart – for Borgers is quite correct in stating that, for Van Ostaijen, theory came after the fact of creation.[7] Only when the tales are seen as a unity, is it possible to deduce the fictional correlative of the Breughel essay. Subsequent pages will deal with various strata of Van Ostaijen's grotesque world in a number of tales. But especially "The Lost House Key" admirably conjoins the general deductions of the essay to a fictional replica.

A synopsis of the plot can be very brief. Hasdrubal Paaltjes, a municipal official, gets drunk one night with some friends. Returning home late at night he finds his house key gone. Paaltjes is unable to enter his house, but he refuses to sleep alone. Aided by the aphrodisiac of champagne, he decides to spend the night with a prostitute. The woman is syphilitic, and Paaltjes contracts the disease. Being an inveterate Don Juan, he spreads it among many women, both married and single. By arithmetical progression, syphilis eventually contaminates the entire city of X, and its way of life becomes geared to a syphilitic *modus vivendi*. Suddenly the reader realizes that this city, now called Megalopolis, has made syphilis the norm and a non-syphilitic existence the anti-norm.

The city is known only as X at the beginning of the story. After the Paaltjesean revolution, it first gains national attention, followed by international fame. The nation to which it belongs severs ties by making it a free city. It becomes a haven for all unwanted human elements from other regions and nations. Social outcasts and outlaws find refuge here. Soon it has achieved status and a name. As Megalopolis it quickly develops features of a city-state. Obviously, city X could never have prospered as Megalopolis does. True, other powers control its foreign policies, but internally it is autonomous. The world powers provide economic aid for Megalopolis, not as a charitable gift, but as an "externally-prophylactic method"; "the existence of this city eliminated venereal diseases, because it concentrated the carriers of this disease in one place." (III, 183) In short, Megalopolis flourishes antithetically. Peccant disorder evolves into the healthy norm. Hence the story may be seen as a symbolization of the grotesque, as the world of absolute *verkeerdheid*.

Insidious relentlessness is equally well exhibited in this tale. A simple, inane mistake catapults a culture into orbit. This phenomenon, observable in other tales, is the grotesque's generating function; an essentially simple incident or rule induces complex patterns. Of course, the tale could be examined from other angles. For example, one could read the story as a vituperative creation of myth. There is the suggestion of a satiric creation-story, which takes evil quite literally in writing its mythical history. On a more general level, the story overthrows ethical morality. An American philosopher remarks at a certain point that Megalopolis had become moral again through immorality. At first the inhabitants were pleased that their peculiar ethics were recognized. "But then they could not understand that it was reduced to a consistent immorality. They laughed at the childish philosophy of the American." (III, 186) A shudder passes through the tale. What up till then might have been a vitriolic satire, now turns into the reality of the grotesque. In a single sentence Van Ostaijen destroys any illusions. "The foundation of Megalopolis was already far in the past." Not only has this luetic civilization attained veracity, but it also has become an historic reality. Even that is not enough. Everyday syphilitic reality has become so mundane and a matter of course that Megalopolis has reached the stage where it can afford wasting effort in society's most sophisticated pastime: arguing about its beginnings.

In this tale we see the rise of a civilization from obscurity to glory. As in other tales, an eccentric progression propels an insignificant negation into a grotesque cosmogony. Inclusiveness anticipates a sense of horror. The rise of Megalopolis is not only inclusive; it might also seem to follow the progressive stages of the city's mythical disease. The primary phase of syphilis is characterized by chancre in the part affected – Paaltjes. The secondary phase spreads to the skin and mucous membranes; rapidly the contagion spreads throughout the city of X. The disease predominates. Luetic Megalopolis is born. The tertiary phase involves the remainder of the body, culminating in infecting the brain. The entire structure and super-structure of Megalopolis has been created. The story ends with senseless debates and wranglings about the question of whether Paaltjes really lost his key or not. Three major factions, psychologists, realists and nominalists, beset each other with obtuse argumentation in a demented fashion, as if the intellect of Megalopolis has been affected by the terminal stage of the disease which founded it. It is no gratuitous accident that Van Ostaijen chose two words which assonate in Dutch (as well as in English). "Syphilis" and "civilization" linguistically and symbolically assimilate to form the implied neologism *syphilization*. This is perhaps the most bitter symbol-ization of Van Ostaijen's nihilistic pessimism.

The symbolic negation of the world by representing it as a luetic organism can be discovered in other tales too. In "Camembert Or the Lucky Lover" for example, there is a condensed version of the metaphoric connotation of "The Lost House Key." Camembert, that most insensate of bourgeois lovers, has been frequenting a brothel with some friends, where he was forcibly ejected because his fear of contracting venereal disease prevented him from consummating his desires. His comrades congratulate him on his stout behavior and exemplary control: "Such characters were the state's best weapon against syphilis." (III, 319) That night he has a morbid dream. He is surrounded by women, whose breasts are transformed into octopuses. "Who vomited syphilis bacilli. Not women overpowered Camembert any-more, but bacilli. His room was filled with them. The world is a great clump. Of syphilis bacilli, naturally. To dream is to rise from petty reality. To be in the universe. Sure." (III, 319) In "Patriotism Incorporated" vene-real contagion again assumes public proportions. In this case, it even becomes a patriotic boon. Pameelke, a cabinet member of Teutonia's government, castigates an international movement for the prevention of venereal disease. Such an institution he finds presumptuous and unethical. Elimination of the disease within national boundaries is the duty of that particular government. However, its presence in another state, such as a neighbouring country, can only give cause for patriotic rejoicing. Venereal contagion in another country means undermining the health and number of its population. A true patriot will laud such a condition, and will heap curses on those who would attempt to eradicate the affliction in nations which are not their native country. The ethical and rhetorical fervor of this vicious reasoning is revolting, and yet consistent with a morally and ethi-cally atrophied society. The individual realms of politics, society and culture in this world of absolute *verkeerdheid* fit the general pattern of inverted, negative, noxious incongruity.

Politics of Corruption

The most obvious thematic constant in these tales is an unremitting critique of the times. The very assiduity of the critique indicates a contemporary world out of joint. Van Ostaijen sees his environment as essentially absurd, and gives artistic expression to his vision through the hypertrophy of the absurdities of normality and the atrophy of common sense-reality. Nothing is sacred. Everything is subject for satire. There are no constants of behavior – moral or psychological. When tabloid reality is a matter of fact despite its horrors, then art can surely posit absurdity as a common denominator of its various manifestations. Daily reality sanctions even the most bizarre artistic inventions. The grotesque is especially pronounced in an era when the dictum "fact is stranger than fiction" is a commonplace. One could conceivably find social and political correlatives for any of the subjects in these tales. A story such as "The Gang of the Trunk" is peopled with scarcely disguised figures from Belgian and French society. The topical significance of the satiric passages has admittedly vanished during the course of time. They could only provide interest now for an historical or sociological study of the Twenties in Belgium. But topicality is minor to a literary consideration of these tales. These stories are not dated *récits à clef,* though at the time their satiric scurrility shocked some people into indignant fury.[8] Their cumulative effect is of primary interest. Furthermore, their mode of vision and artistic expression places them within the mainstream of modern fiction. Even their themes are familiar echoes to present literary and factual experience.

The protest against modern times embraces the political, sociological and cultural aspects of society. Van Ostaijen experienced the First World War at home in Antwerp as a citizen of the Belgian nation. He suffered from its political and economic aftermath in Berlin, where he witnessed revolution in the streets and the impact of inflation. Van Ostaijen lived in an era which saw practically everything of the old order vanish in a series of momentous political, economic, intellectual, scientific and artistic revolutions. He reflects most of these upheavals in his tales. The world in which he lived and the world which he created are equally sinister and uncanny. In these tales there is little comfort for the victims of a grotesque order.

The characters fear life and not death. The inability to control events instills a paralyzing feeling of impotence. Laughter is one of the few defenses against such a monolithic absurdity.

But the laughter is bitter and gives no release. The other defense, as a later chapter will point out, is art. Art remains the only constant. It is an art that turns away from reality to establish an expression which abstracts experience into formulations alien to traditional preconceptions. What then are the components of a world created from such negative reactions?

The tale "Patriotism Incorporated" opens with the short liturgical phrase: "In illo tempore." What are these fictional times which, as all grotesques do, mirror an existing order to a certain degree? Pameelke, the cabinet minister, can only report anarchy, upheavals and aberrations of the reactionary norm. But what Pameelke's diagnosis of the political situation calls a "madhouse," refers in reality to certain movements which attempt to forestall another world war and try to instill a sense of reason in those nations that formerly settled their differences through war. Pameelke's indignation concerns internationalists, the League of Nations, and any other institution which would prevent a political system from throwing the world into another cataclysm. Pameelke and his confederates want to uphold the old order. The old order managed to keep the masses ignorant of political facts, and roused their spirits with slogans of patriotism, monarchy, and the essentially evil nature of any nation other than their own.

Here again one finds the double-edged sword of Van Ostaijen's grotesque fiction. What Pameelke fears are exactly those ideas which might save Europe from future disasters. His diagnosis of Europe is pertinent, except that what he considers the cure is really the disease. These are bad times, feels Pameelke. The masses are losing their blind faith in authority. A strong feeling of internationalism is growing, which tries to prevent the dangerous excesses of nationalism. And nationalism is the main instigator of wars. Wars are the backbone of national economies. Therefore internationalism and the people's disregard for patriotic inducements for war will be disastrous. Something needs to be done. The savior is Dr. Erich-Carl Wybau. Wybau is totally amoral, apolitical and a consequent pessimist. Nothing has superior relevance for him. Ideas are inherently nonsense. For this extreme sceptic, the only category in life is "doing." The result of the "doing" is totally irrelevant. Wybau sees existence as empty and meaningless. The function of his life is filling his existence, occupying himself, even if it is only make-believe. For Wybau everything is relative – even relativity. In his lengthy argumentation, Wybau prescribes a cure for the disease that is posing a threat to national prosperity.

He postulates, first, that as leaders they are entirely different from and superior to the masses they rule. The masses believe in slogans which are essentially lies. But the leaders must face facts and realize that *all* slogans are relative and meaningless. It takes him little trouble to convince them of their primary desire – to be boss. Once they are the masters of their country, they only desire the supremacy of that nation. This implies complete control over the masses. To obtain complete control is to unite the people behind their sentiment of patriotism. But the patriotism of the masses is realistic and not idealistic. The cause must be "right." To find the right cause is easy. Just present the national cause as one of absolute right. It is an illusion in most cases, but that is irrelevant. What the leaders know has nothing to do with what they proclaim in public. The illusion of righteousness is all-important. Once it has been established that absolute right is a patriotic affair, all that is left is to rouse the masses and make them feel that they are fighting for an absolute right. This can only be brought about by having the neighbouring country's government (Fochany) be guilty of violating that absolute right. In such a case Teutonia has the illusion of defense, and the people will blindly follow any suggestion of their leaders. The logical conclusion of the argument is that patriotism is needed, and that it is needed by all nations.

Chauvinism, therefore, is an international affair. Wybau proposes to borrow the methods of the internationalists in establishing an international organization for the propagation of chauvinism. For every nation will surely realize that patriotism cannot be a one-sided affair. It has to exist on both sides of the border, otherwise it is meaningless and doomed to failure. Since in this particular instance they are primarily concerned with the rivalry between Teutonia and Fochany, he announces the formation of a "Fochano-Teutonic Company for the Exploitation of Patriotism." The motto of Patriotism Incorporated will be "Chauvinists of all nations, unite!"

Given the situation, the results are predictable. Fochany also sees the need for chauvinism since its government, too, is losing control over the masses. The company is formed. With the usual methods of insinuation, "incidents," false reportage, governmental covering-up, the patriotic citizens of the two nations are soon roused. Mobilization is required. Military needs are to be fulfilled, and the economy gets into gear again. The company, like all companies, holds its annual meeting. They all agree that everything is going well. The leaders of the rival countries toast each other's health. Someone at the meeting hints at a false note during the merriment by suggesting that, since both nations have strong patriotic populations again, have large armies and flourishing economies, the need of the Trust is no longer warranted. But Wybau saves the day again. He argues that it is precisely in wartime that the Trust is of extreme importance. The Trust can lengthen or shorten wars according to the wishes of the trustees. It can also regulate the end of wars, so that the losing government will not be threatened by a revolution, but will be able to remain in office. For it is to the advantage of the partner, who is the ostensible enemy, to have the vanquished nation on its feet again as soon as possible. Hence, orates Wybau, the Trust is above the vicissitudes of war and peace, and controls "eternally" "the fate of Europe." It should be the nation's "metaphysic." With consistent logic, a principally negative inversion of reality has reached the status of an absolute.

Van Ostaijen ends the story with a final twist. The grotesque logic of an unprincipled sceptic enjoys its ultimate triumph. Theory has become reality. The "Neiffeltower" in Fochany has been stolen. The capital of Fochany is in an uproar, and the population agrees with the newspapers that, obviously, Teutonia must have perpetrated this crime. Wybau and Pameelke are taking a stroll through Fochany's capital after the annual meeting of the Trust has ajourned. Pameelke suddenly exclaims that the Neiffeltower is still there, that it was not stolen at all. Wybau tells him to keep quiet; people might otherwise hear him and take up his cry. The people are standing in droves in front of the Neiffeltower screaming that the building has been stolen by the Teutonians. The telegraph-operators on top are busily sending messages across the world that the Teutonians have stolen the tower they are transmitting from. Reality is totally powerless.

"In illo tempore" we find a totally corrupt political system, unprincipled in a consistent fashion and bent on individual gain. Europe is ruled by either unscrupulous and stupid officials or by unprincipled, amoral men like Wybau. The masses are the ignorant and gullible plebs, easily fooled and loyal to their folly. This is a situation of organic folly, which is at the core of the world. Nothing can be done about it. A note of desperate frustration can be heard in Pameelke's first speech. It is quite obvious that Van Ostaijen thoroughly agrees with Pameelke's exhortations that the world is a madhouse. He is also clearly on the side of the rehabilitating forces of which Pameelke is afraid. But in order to bring the truth home, he depicts a world gone quite mad. And in this world one cannot hold the Wybaus responsible. Wybau is a totally unscrupulous and pessimistic sceptic, taking advantage of a sick world by prescribing the medicine it wants to have, although it will not cure but aggravate the insalubrious condition. He merely carries the known factor of madness to its logical extreme. It is a world where thought is "crippled by a stupid logic." (III, 85) Wybau accepts this premise, and brilliantly argues the basic stupidity into accepted reality.

The world depicted in "Patriotism Incorporated" is a norm for all passages where the political climate is revealed. An inhuman system with no redemptive qualities, it is an immediate reflection of a disordered world. The political system is totally corrupt, and yet it feels that it is being assailed by forces which, from its standpoint, are revolutionary and irrational. In "The Prison in Heaven" one finds a similar political situation. The masses have been clamoring for individual freedom from the subordination of corporate institutions such as Church and State. At this moment of crisis "No. 200," the released prisoner who cannot live in freedom but is haunted by his "will-to-prison," comes as a godsend. Very quickly, he is advertised as an example of the fact that individual freedom is an act of treason against Church and State. The priest who tours the country with No. 200 in a sideshow argues that the jailbird carries freedom within his soul yet hankers to be voluntarily imprisoned. Prison, he argues is "a function of the state and religion." To go voluntarily to prison is to "praise God and the King." "This simple jailbird has recognized that prison has a necessary function in the state." There is no higher freedom than to go voluntarily to prison. (III, 132)

This justification for a totalitarian state echoes a phrase in "Patriotism Incorporated." "But a free people must realize that freedom is the highest good a free people can possess, worth sacrificing all your freedom for, and worth defending to your last breath. It goes without saying that concrete freedom must always be sacrificed to the abstract, the moral freedom." (III, 49) There is another parallel between "Patriotism Incorporated" and "The Prison in Heaven." In the latter tale the political system is also represented as a corporation, "Religion, Morality, State and Co." There is no anti-trust law in this world of corporate folly.

Because of No. 200, things are running smoothly again for the State. The masses (as in "Patriotism Incorporated") have been successfully brain-washed by the advertising campaign of State and Church. The entire society succumbs to the official argument that real freedom lies in a voluntary prison sentence. "Never did the royal house stand on a foundation of such solid citizen loyalty as at this time. Religion flourished; many Masses were said for the peace of souls, births and abortions." (III, 133) Fallacy has again become truth. But No. 200, the consistent idealist of the "will-to-prison," finds his present stardom not answering to his ideal demands. He does not want to live in an artificially simulated prison-existence. He wants to be in a real prison; he is consequent and adamant. But inside a prison he is of little use to the authorities. No. 200 decides to force the issue. He kills the priest in whose show he toured the nation. Although he commits the crime in full view of the crowd, and although he surrenders voluntarily, no one wants to arrest him. But his crime is, nevertheless, cataclysmic for the State and Church Inc. He has commited a crime against the State and the Church, so by law he must die. He is no good to them in prison, and yet they cannot let him go free. People are already clamoring to know why No. 200 could not go to prison if he desired it so fervently. It is decided that No. 200 committed treason and must die, if only to save the authorities from embarrassment. But death is not what he bargained for. No. 200 considers the penalty of death a miscarriage of justice. All he ever asked for was a life sentence.

With the cooperation of the prison chaplain, the Church and State attempt to profit from No. 200's death and to rectify, to some degree, the upheaval his action has caused. The lengthy argument of the chaplain can be condensed as follows. If he, No. 200, would cry out, "I deserved this," when he is going to be beheaded, he would be reinstituting the honor of Church, State and Monarchy. He would thereby also assure himself his most fervent wish, an eternal prison in heaven. No. 200 agrees, and the chaplain writes him a "physical-metaphysical check" from his checkbook, "Good for ONE (1) PRISON IN HEAVEN." (III, 139) Now everything should be all right again. No. 200's admission of guilt should bring the masses back under control. But he muffs his cue. In order to make sure that the crowd, surprised upon hearing his declaration, should understand what it means, he cries out: "I have earned it, the prison in heaven." (III, 140) In this world of deceit and corrupt systems, an innocent idealist had the last word, though being cheated in advance.

In most of the tales some element of politics is burlesqued. But there is one story completely devoted to the political machinery. In "Splendor and Decline of a Politician" ("Glans en verval van een politiek man") Mr. Visschers, a talented politician with a great future in the liberal party, patiently waits for the death of three party members who are ahead of him in seniority. While he waits over the years, the party's popularity declines. When the last of his rivals has finally died, the party does not exist any longer. By this time Mr. Visschers himself is no longer recognized by the man in the street. A waitress tells him the story of Mr. Visscher's life without realizing to whom she is talking. Under the quiet, even surface of the story lies the frustration already noted in other tales. It cannot find release in action. At the end of the story Mr. Visschers is not only incapable of action, but is also impotent. The tale represents the political system as a ruthless anomaly. Mr. Visschers wishes his seniors dead without any moral compunction. The system itself, the party, pays no attention to a talented man, whom it slowly destroys. As in the other stories, an inhuman and relentless force plays with the destiny of an individual. Ruthless circumstances are beyond the control of the individual. Circumstances reduce him to impotence, incapacity of action and frustration.

Economics of Inflation

In the collection of *jeux de mots* or *jeux d'esprit* called *The Zoo for Children of Our Time*, is a piece one-and-a-half sentence long. "The plover is a bird which lays expensive eggs. In countries with a poor rate of exchange the plover no longer lays any eggs." (III, 236) Uyttersprot points out that plover eggs were a delicacy in Germany and very expensive. He also notes that in 1923 Germany was being ruined by inflation.[9] This theme of inflation is the subject of the story "The Adventures of Mercurius, Corporation for the Exploitation of Counterfeiting." Employing the same principle as in the other stories, Van Ostaijen presents an inverted world, where inflation is a *conditio sina qua non* and counterfeiting a honorable business. The theme of corporate institutions also recurs. The counterfeiters see their occupation as a serious business proposition. In order to survive the vicissitudes of the economy, they propose to form a company, since "only forming a trust can save us." Van Ostaijen gives a hint in this story as to why he sees the modern world as a grotesque corporate venture. The counterfeiters are proud of their decision, because the act of forming a trust provides their venture with scientific dignity.

The definition of "The Plover" is a succinct thematic summation of the longer story. The counterfeit bills are equal to the plover eggs, while counterfeiting is the plover. And the plover cannot lay eggs in countries where inflation has ruined the economy. Counterfeiting is a conservative business; it can only have profitable results in nations with a stable economy. The company for the exploitation of counterfeiting is prone to fail because of the world's irrationality. Reality dooms their venture. The thousand-mark bills they produce are absolutely perfect, but in order to obtain this perfection, too much time has to pass. In the interim period the mark has dropped still further, and the real as well as counterfeit thousand-mark bills are worthless. Harassed by the anger of one of the partners, Süsswein, himself a partner and the company's production manager, becomes desperate. Trying to offset the losses, he uses bad paper to produce hundred-thousand mark bills more quickly. Since the quality of the product is bad, the group is almost immediately arrested. Their sentences are heavy. Süsswein's lawyer pleads innocent. He argues that under inflationary conditions, counterfeiting is an act of philanthrophy since Süsswein wanted merely to alleviate the shortage of the national treasury. Süsswein is an idealist. He recognizes this position when he tells the court that he is glad to go to prison, since reality has already punished him enough. In the present state of the nation and national economy, it is an unrewarding occupation to be a counterfeiter. The struggle for life is becoming increasingly difficult. To be a criminal is a better social standing than being a counterfeiter. Reality is absurd, and vice is virtue.

Inflation and jazz are the stars of Van Ostaijen's projected film "Bankruptcy Jazz." The film would have depicted a totally chaotic world, where national bankruptcy is the rule and Charlie Chaplin the head of state. (III, 286) Frenetic jazz music (Dixieland at the time) represents a civilization which has erupted into total anarchy. The Dada movement and national governments work hand in hand. The new national hymn is the conjugation of *Ich bin pleite, Du bist pleite, etc.* (III, 288) "Bankruptcy Jazz" pictures the total madness which stories like "Patriotism Incorporated" and "The adventures of Mercurius" hint at in a less abrasive manner.

Warfare as a Platonic Ideal

Inversions of normality – the will-to-prison versus freedom, counterfeiting versus legal tender, chauvinism versus internationalism – become the norm and are enforced with a perverse legality. The effect of *Verfremdung* is only enhanced when in this inverted world the metastasis of ordinary existence becomes an ideal, a supreme achievement. Another example of this principle is the military system in these grotesques. War had become a major political, social and artistic issue during and after the First World War. The political system of Van Ostaijen's grotesque world sees warfare as the ultimate goal for a nation. War is imperative from the point of view of the politician in "Patriotism Incorporated." Pameelke insists that from an economic point of view, war is a state of perfection. Grotesque logic reasons this premise to its absurd conclusion in "The General." The exiled Peruvian General, Ricardo Gomes, postulates "pure war" or "true martiality." War as it is waged these days is, he feels, but a sorry approximation of what it really should be. In this lengthy and closely reasoned tale, Van Ostaijen builds a fantastic case for pure martiality and man's basically warlike nature. Man is born with the desire for war in his blood. His childhood games are all warlike. This warlike urge in man's subconscious is the only true form of martiality. But in our modern society we mistake militarism for true warfare. According to the principles of absurd reasoning, outlined in the subsequent chapter on style, the *idea* of war is reasoned to its ultimate conclusion. There is such a thing as paradigmatic war. War is an ideal, a spiritual necessity.[10] Once this is established, the stage is set for the final absurd twist.

The true basis for war is eroticism, postulates the General. Eroticism is the common denominator of mankind. Hence it follows logically that modern armies should be formed according to the principles of man's erotic nature. The General proceeds to unfold his blueprint for the ideal army. He would divide an army into regiments of homosexuals, sadists, masochists, fetishists and heterosexuals. The General's theory is based on Plato's definition of Eros as a spiritual force which longs to reach the ideality of paradigmatic love. Eros is a metaphysical force because of its transcendental longing. Eroticism is the sexual realization of Eros. Ergo, eroticism is the only basis for waging war in the true spirit of pure martiality. The argument is supported by appealing to the best of man's culture. The narrator is a poet. To convince him, the General uses the analogy of bourgeois art as opposed to true art – i.e. militarism versus pure martiality. Waging war, from the General's point of view, is like the act of creation for the artist. Plato's philosophy of Eros as a spiritual force which reaches for the paradigmatic One, postulates for the General that war is the supreme expression of spiritual man. In fact, Plato is invoked at various points in the narrative. The fanatic soldier is a Platonic idealist. Such a condition is grotesque to be sure. But the *persiflage* is quite serious. Again, Van Ostaijen has merely carried an existing phenomenon in the world of reality to its logical extreme. If Western society insists that war is inevitable, Van Ostaijen appears to be saying, then war should be treated as a basic factor in man's existence. In the world of the grotesque, war has reached the level of being the most supreme expression of Western culture.

The choice of eroticism as the ideal basis of waging war is equally pertinent to the times. Freud and his theory that sexuality is the psychological condition of mankind had obtained prominence during the Twenties. Freudian sexual theory was particularly repugnant to Van Ostaijen. In several tales he attacks Freudianism and psychoanalysis in his usual fashion; he agrees with Freud that sex is the basis for human behavior and proceeds to reason it into absurdity. Only indirectly does Van Ostaijen exercise critical judgment in "The General." The General does his best thinking when he is inebriated. The implication is obvious. The lengthy explanations of his theory that war equals eros are the product of an intoxicated mind.

Secondly, the General commits suicide. Stated parenthetically, this fact goes almost unnoticed. However, the suicide indicates complete disillusion and negates, from a psychological point of view, the veracity of the argument.

In "Hierarchy" militarism is satirized more venomously. In this story three major features of Van Ostaijen's grotesque world are assailed: militarism, sexuality and social hierarchy. An army unit is holding the town of Cataro. They face a grave problem. Soldiers need sexual release. But there are hardly any women in Cataro, nor is there a public brothel. A local citizen solves the problem. He finds four women and a house. One great difficulty still faces him, the military hierarchy of rank. With the little he has at his disposal, he proposes a brilliant solution. In the four rooms of the house he places a couch and a bed. The bed is for officers, the couch for enlisted men. Military hierarchy has been preserved and discipline maintained. The civilian is awarded the title "engineer of erotic affairs." (III, 396) Despite such admirable discipline, this army is subsequently defeated. With one sentence Van Ostaijen generalizes this inhuman microcosmos: "Cataro brothel, myth of our civilization!"

The political structure of Van Ostaijen's grotesque world is corrupt, materialistic, inhuman and tyrannical. Individual freedom is a threat against the state, and needs to be eliminated. The state as an ideal does not exist. Individual politicians in league with monarchies are either ignorant or unprincipled; all are corrupt. The ruling class is only interested in maintaining a profitable situation for personal gain at the cost of a nation's population. The masses are no serious threat to their reactionary principles. People are easily persuaded, fickle, gullible and uncritical of slogans. No one questions the insistence that war is inevitable and that it is the backbone of national economies. The social and political world is a monolithic evil. Individuals are impotent and frustrated. They are incapable of action. The sheer force of circumstances crushes all individual attempts at asserting freedom of action. The symbol for this organized monolith is the corporation. The state is a corporate institution run by a board of corrupt trustees. This is organized chaos. Inflation wrecks the economy. Bellicose patriotism is agitated to ensure wars. War is a fundamental condition of Western civilization.

The Bourgeois as the Perfect Grotesque Citizen

Van Ostaijen singles out three specific nations which, he feels, exhibit particular features of the grotesque world. Germany in particular is criticized in "Hierarchy," "The Adventures of Mercurius," "Patriotism Incorporated," "Bankruptcy Jazz" and in "The German" ("De Duitser");

France in "The Gang of the Trunk" and in "Patriotism Incorporated"; Belgium is attacked in just about all the stories which criticize social or political elements. Under the name of Atupal, a palindrome for Swift's *Laputa,* it is specifically burlesqued in "The Gang of the Trunk" and "The Poet's Profession" ("Het beroep van de dichter"). The social and political structures in most of the tales are a caricature of Belgian society. However, Van Ostaijen uses specific conditions only as details for a general, universal picture of consistent incongruity. That picture presents the grotesque world as diseased. The element of frustration and horror in Van Ostaijen's pessimism comes from the realization that there is no cure for this sick world. On the contrary, it has made itself invincible by organizing itself. Political, economic and military strata of this grotesque society are each corrupt in their own way. The question arises: What sort of people inhabit this world? Van Ostaijen is quite adamant in his answer. The bourgeois is the perfect citizen of the world of the grotesque.

The grotesque, however, does not allow the bourgeois to enjoy a sense of security. In these tales, Van Ostaijen wages a relentless battle against him. Van Ostaijen's weapons are exactly those elements which the bourgeois fears or relies on: the irrational, the incongruous, the discords of existence. The bourgeois champions the ordinary, the normal, the common, the order of laws and regulations. Van Ostaijen denies him his customary sanctuary or subverts it. Perhaps it is Van Ostaijen's ultimate triumph to formulate a grotesque world on bourgeois principles. Collectively, these tales might be interpreted as a vociferous anti-bourgeois critique. The criticism is not concentrated in a single fictional unit, but distributed among the tales. Since this is an examination of the tales as a unified body of work, there has been no attempt to explore each story for every possible detail critical of bourgeois society. What follows is a composite picture, and a negative one.

The prototype of the bourgeois depicted in these tales is the public notary Telleke. Telleke is the hero of two short tales. In "The Money-Box" ("De Cassette") Telleke has become the proud owner of a small safe. Only he knows the combination. Telleke feels absolutely secure about the safety of his family's valuables. His safe becomes to him the symbol of security: an absolute. One day the safe disappears. Telleke and other local notables cannot accept the fact of theft. It is against the norm. Safes with secret combinations are made to be opened and not for taking away. If this is not so, what point is there in acquiring a safe with a secret combination? That is to say, a norm cannot be abnormal. In the case of Telleke we might rephrase this; a norm has *no right* to be abnormal. The incongruous has no legitimate right in a well-ordered society. "We are used to having money-boxes ransacked, but to carry money-boxes away is an anarchical principle. Proceeding from this, what form of self-defense would remain for solid citizens?" (III, 171) Even when they finally accept the possibility of theft, incongruity persists. What possible good can a safe be to a thief who does not know the secret combination? But this last vestige of reason is negated by the discovery of the safe, broken open, on a country road. The subject of the tale is simple and ludicrous. But its thematic implications hold true for most of the tales. In the bourgeois world order is an imperative. It cannot tolerate violation of an axiomatic code. In this case, safes have a specific principle (i.e., safes are theft-proof) which may not be violated. When it is, a world is suddenly fearfully alienated. In Van Ostaijen's grotesques the most mundane becomes preposterously charged with the absurd.

"The Money-Box" also implies the inability of the bourgeois to perceive nuances. His dogmatic adherence to an authorized certainty cannot allow ambivalence, modifications or nuances. The middle-class man is intellectually and spiritually blind. To maintain order he will rely on logic. His opinions are documented, and proof provides authority. Van Ostaijen simply pursues this authority to its unreasonable extreme. For example, Telleke is convinced that speed causes accidents. In "The Conviction of Notary Telleke" he substantiates his conviction with the observation that if someone places one foot too quickly in front of the other, he will fall. Urged on by his friends, he takes an express train. His friends have not convinced him, but Telleke has agreed to take the risk. Once inside the train, his conviction that speed equals disaster frightens him. The uncertainty whether there will be an accident or not is his undoing. Telleke, with a logic typical for Van Ostaijen in these tales, follows his conviction to its absurd extreme; to prevent disaster, he jumps out of the window of the speeding train. At that moment he realizes that the absurd won. "Even my most extreme effort to evade the accident was of no use." (III, 173) The expected never did materialize. Telleke thought to save himself by his preventive action only to find that his reasoning resulted in a negative conclusion.[11]

Telleke fears suspension in uncertainty. In the world of the grotesque there is no certainty except that of the existence of the absurd itself. The bourgeois has lost his footing. He has lost the sanctuary of his ordered reality. As Christian Morgenstern pointed out, "Unter bürgerlich verstehe ich das, worin sich der Mensch bisher geborgen gefühlt hat." Morgenstern's etymology derives Bürger from Burg, a derivative of the verb bergen (to shield, shelter, harbor).[12] Van Ostaijen removes this traditional shelter of authority, security, sanctity. The bourgeois is no longer geborgen but very vulnerable. Throughout the tales Van Ostaijen strips bourgeois society of its snug sanctuaries. But he cannot rid the world of the bourgeois.

"The Gang of the Trunk" inverts social mores with assiduous vengeance. The tale's milieu is admittedly not specifically bourgeois. Its background is the world of aristocrats, on the one hand, and the world of criminals on the other. However, appearances are always deceiving in these tales. Little Comtesse Angèle is the typical example of the preconception of a charming and innocent girl indigent to the popular novel. She has been educated and raised in a convent school. She is the product of respectability and correct breeding. High society regards her as a charming *ingénue*. Everyone is somewhat astounded when she becomes engaged to the Marquis de Mirlitonare. To all the eligible notables it seems a strange choice to pick a man who has no legs: the marquis walks on artificial limbs. But little Angèle is apparently completely infatuated with her lover. Before the marriage can take place, a gang of criminals kidnaps the Marquis and substitutes one of its own group. Alessandro is also a truncated man and from the same country as the real Marquis. Here we can ascertain again how in the grotesque world of Van Ostaijen established hierarchy has little meaning. The petty criminal Alessandro and the nobleman de Mirlitonare are like two drops of water. Only the "brains" of the gang, Dr. Knackfuss, perceives some slight physical differences, physiognomic nuances, as it were: the nose, the lips and the length of the stumps are not identical. But a small operation performed by Dr. Knackfuss will obliterate these slight differences, and transplant the Roman nose of the Marquis to Alessandro's face. In agriculture, Knackfuss is careful to point out, such a process of grafting is called a proces of ennobling. Social distinctions are a matter of degree, of nuance; the exchange of a plebeian for an artistocratic nose makes a nobleman out of criminal.

Van Ostaijen emphasizes this similarity ostensibly for purposes of plot. But his intentions can not be mistaken. "Also pure chance that the truncated maquereau and the truncated Marquis resembled each other like twins. But the Marquis was a little more trunk; that's why he had one syllable less. All pure chance." (III, 68) Social distinctions have been negated by making them subject to a mere interchange of physical and rather inconsequential properties. Grotesque equality enforces absurd neutrality. Knackfuss makes the point quite clear to the captured Marquis. The only difference between him and his prisoner is a matter of social level. But this is not a qualitative difference, merely a difference of milieux. And this, as was shown, has little real significance. Knackfuss summarizes his argument with the succinct adage: "You play with the white pawns, and I with the black ones. That is all." (III, 81) In chess, the advantage of playing with white rather than black is a matter of chance.

In the world of absolute *verkeerdheid* a pimp is the equal of a marquis. Angèle, the model debutante, turns out to be not only devious, but also a pathological case of sexual deviation. In the person of Angèle, marital infidelity and nymphomania are carried to their extreme. The bourgeois sanctity of marriage has become a hollow phrase. Coincidentally, Alessandro, who thought to reap the fruits of the fraud, is now its victim. For Angèle has purposely married a truncated man. Her husband must be powerless to act, but may not be impotent. For she can only attain sexual satisfaction by committing adultery in the presence of her husband. Angèle has her own perverse absolute; a husband is an archetypal fool, nevertheless, he must play his customary role. It is, no matter how immoral, a game with strict rules. Similarly, Angèle has her own stringent morality. It is beneath her, for example, to betray her husband behind his back. "To be unfaithful behind his back was too common for Angèle. A Countess Collin is unfaithful in a courtly fashion, when the spouse is present." (III, 93) Alessandro has become a fetish and, as a husband, a mere decorative symbol. Given the inverse of normality, Angèle insists that it is bourgeois to betray her husband with only one man. "It was not in keeping with the erotic determination of the Marquise to betray her husband in a scandalously bourgeois manner with only *one* third party, nor to affirm such a relationship as a domestic matter of course. The man in the fool's costume had to play his role in front of many lovers. Making him ridiculous by means of merely one relationship was not worthy of the Marquise, but only of girl friends from the convent school who came from a bourgeois tradition." (III, 101) Not only Knackfuss and other members of the gang are invited to Angèle's bed, but also teenagers from a local high school and many others. To underscore the decorative function of the husband, Alessandro is placed on a pedestal every night to preside, as it were, over the infidelity of his wife. Absurdity knows no extremes. Angèle persists in maintaining the invere legality of the husband's hierarchal rights as head of the family by asking him to choose a lover for her that night. His word is law. She tells him that she, the slave of his command, wallows in immorality to serve his decorative supremacy. Even when Alessandro confesses to the fraud nothing changes. He sadly reflects that the prostitutes for whom he used to be a sexual talisman were purer than the countess he is married to. The processes of the incongruous have attained their goal. In this world of consequent incongruity prostitutes are, if not superior, at least equal to countesses.

Despite the scurrility of the plot, "The Gang of the Trunk" is written in the same stylized language as the other tales. A subsequent discussion of "Ika Loch's Brothel" will point out that subject matter does not influence the style in a drastic manner. The very pounderousness of the style neutralizes the most "shocking" subject matter. In the case of "The Gang of the Trunk," Van Ostaijen does play some stylistic tricks however. He parodies the stale verbosity and cliché-ridden prose of popular potboilers. Thematically, the story parodies the romantic dime novel. The criminals are inverted stereotypes. The criminal hero Alessandro is a good-natured cripple. The young heroine, equipped with all the usual trappings of beauty, youth, innocence and aristocracy, reveals herself as a sadistic and masochistic adulteress. Notice the absence of tragedy, pathos or even bathos. Angèle's sexual aberration is an intellectual deviation from the romantic norm. "The Gang of the Trunk" negates the traditional bourgeois sanctities of society, matrimony, conjugal rights, romantic love – indeed of romanticism itself.

In the opening paragraph of "Claire's Herd" Van Ostaijen subtly, by means of an almost mathematical progression of associations, describes the dissolution of a bourgeois marriage. The husband is too busy with his business affairs, and feels entitled after eighteen years of marriage to try, as he puts it euphemistically, "other possibilities in life." (III, 290) The wife, playing the familiar game of a woman's age being a progression of diminishing returns, seeks the company of young Don Juans. However, the narrator assures us, there is no proof of actual adultery on either side. The passage is a masterpiece of innuendo, told with sobriety and slyly constrained mockery. This introduction to "Claire's Herd" follows a familiar pattern. Setting out to be a harmless explanation of why their eighteen-year-old daughter Claire is no longer restricted to parental control, it unobtrusively develops into an argument to disclose the reasons for the parents' alleged mutual infidelity. This, in turn, undermines through innuendo and implication the very situation it set out to justify. In "The Kept Hotel Key" the wife sweetly condones her husband's drunken escapades – as long as he doesn't become involved with "strange women." The truth of the matter is that the husband both drinks to excess and frequents every brothel he can find.

Each tale contains details which indict specific aspects of bourgeois society. They are too numerous to be included here. Only a few more instances may suffice. The theme of monolithic society can also be found in "A Fatality" ("Een fataliteit"). The hero is again a bourgeois, in this case a *nouveau riche*. Money elevates him from a shabby apartment to a mansion in the wealthy section of town. His wife is no longer fat, while his daughters can only be approached by young men holding at least the rank of lieutenant. But this pillar of society is the victim of its strong sense of hierarchy. The family carries a stigma which is slowly undermining his health and sanity: his surname is Purée.[13]

"Camembert Or The Lucky Lover" portrays a bourgeois Don Juan. Camembert is the *non plus ultra* of the common man and the most commonplace, boring lover imaginable. Circumstances propel him into prominence as a lover, making him a famous Don Juan by default. Self-satisfied, sedate and utterly complacent, his erotic life-cycle conforms to the norm. Camembert justifies everything that happens to him by means of his imperturbable complacency. Once he was, through no fault of his own, the dashing young lover for whom *demi-mondaines* kept rich old gentlemen waiting in their closets. When Camembert is a rich old gentleman himself, he must undergo the same humiliation, yet he does not see any correlation. He feels no remorse, no anger. Camembert knows no passion. He is the symbol of self-satisfied mediocrity. Life happens to him, but it effects no change. Passionless, common and mediocre, Camembert is the bourgeois who has killed romanticism.

No other tale sums up Van Ostaijen's dislike of bourgeois society in quite so vituperative a fashion as the page-and-a-half "History" ("Geschiedenis"). The anonymity of the title extends to the tale itself, for not one of the characters has a name. In this way Van Ostaijen extends his criticism to an entire civilization in an almost allegorical manner. These shorter pieces do not have the usual stylistic or argumentative digressions to undermine the story-line. Their satiric tension is not refracted. But like the other and longer tales, they do not have a cathartic conclusion either.

In "History" Van Ostaijen's nihilistic sense of life is presented almost schematically. Wealth and social status are represented by a distinguished-*looking* pederast, who distributes empty candy-boxes to boys on the street only after he has eaten all the bonbons. Though the youths worship him, his beneficence is obviously only illusory. This does not prevent them from ascribing unquestionable authority to him on the mere strength of his appearance. A gentleman who "looked less distinguished" tells the distinguished-looking gentleman to give the youths candy instead of empty boxes. Authority is outraged. The distinguished-looking gentleman calls the other a traitor and a Jew, and stands by in righteous indignation while the youths beat the less distinguished-looking gentleman to death. Even when the unfortunate idealist explains to the mob that he is working in their behalf, they will not believe him. Appearances are reality. They have a simple and undeniable proof of his villainy and of the other gentleman's integrity; "We know a gentleman with a top hat is a distinguished gentleman. He has our welfare at heart." (III, 146) The symbol of reasonable reality is denied any verisimilitude at all by the grotesque. Not only is the less distinguished-looking gentleman murdered, but his corpse is so mutilated that the municipal morgue refuses to accept it since it can not be proven that it was a human body. The next day the distinguished-looking gentlemen performs exactly the same rite, except that he adds one bonbon for each youth as a bonus. Their gratitude for his magnanimity knows no bounds. He modestly declines all praise with the sententious remark that the proverb tells one to do good. To prove his sympathy he rapes a small boy.

This short tale is a good example of Van Ostaijen's bitterness toward society, the bourgeois and the world he lived in. External factors distinguish people from each other in a totally arbitrary manner. Hierarchy must be strictly maintained despite proof of its utter absurdity. The authority spawned by this corrupt society is blindly followed, and shows its gratitude for this trust by desecration. Idealism has absolutely no meaning in this world, and, if necessary, it will even be eradicated. Traditional authority is amoral, sinister and dangerous. Social standing is hollow and based on totally meaningless distinctions. This is a grim and bleak world of absolute power which brooks no discontent.

Art as a Grotesque Irrelevancy

Van Ostaijen's substitute cosmos of the grotesque also includes a cultural or artistic stratum. Being an artist himself, it is understandable that Van Ostaijen did not preserve a distancing in his treatment of this subject equal to other topics, such as politics or the social hierarchy. Nevertheless, its inclusion in the topography of the grotesque world merits brief examination. Van Ostaijen never enjoyed commercial success as an artist. He stitched his livelihood together from various literary activities, odd jobs, and, especially in Berlin, from personal loans. It seems, therefore, only logical to find pecuniary aid to the artist as the subject of the little sketch "Portrait of a Young Maecenas" ("Portret van een jonge maeceen").[14]

This tale discovers an *a priori* condition of want for the artist. Deprivation is maintained by the bourgeoisie with the aid of the critics. Following a familiar pattern of reasoning, impecuniosity is not imposed on artists for any spiteful reason, but merely for their own advantage. "That's why all artists go hungry. Because society wants to preserve their powers of creativity. It is completely wrong to believe that society is not concerned about artists. On the contrary. It will even go so far as to admit to the sad necessity of a negative role for itself in order to create sufficient opportunity for developing the positive force." The old argument that an artist must suffer in order to create is applied with a vengeance. In the artistic as well as in all the other strata of the grotesque world, classification is a morbid obsession. It is the incorporation of authority through systematization, and it seems to cast a spell of infallibility and permanence. Hungry artists, for example, are classified according to two types: tame and flamboyant ones. The world of the Maecenas is equally categorized. A young Maecenas is different from an older, more accomplished one. "There are many Maecenases. That's why one must specialize." The more inept, "less stereotyped" version of the philanthropic species finds his *raison d'être* in all the platitudes so familiar in "enlightened" circles of bourgeois society. Art can not really be paid in proportion to its timeless value. The non-artist is morally bound to recognize the unique phenomenon of the artist and must care for him as if he were a hothouse plant. The young Maecenas glories in his professional insignificance.

The result of these noble sentiments is a fraudulent business venture. The Maecenas buys canvases on the basis of friendship, which implies friendly prices. His generosity includes cigarettes and profitable transactions. Since art cannot be proportionally rewarded, it follows only logically that 100 in payment for a work of art is the same as 10,000. "It really remains just as far from the absolute value of art." The young Maecenas feels superior to other patrons of the arts. Others simply buy, and think that thereby their obligation has been fulfilled. But the young Maecenas is superior to these mundane spirits since he truly appreciates art and, correlatively, knows himself eternally on its debit side. Naturally this does not prevent him from paying as little as possible. His guilt makes up the difference. The young Maecenas wallows voluptuously in guilt. "To confess to his bad conscience is for him a gentle coitus. That's why he wants to remain eternally indebted to the artists, in order to preserve this coitus." The grotesque magician's trick, which makes normal, essential truths disappear behind trivialities or behind absolute folly, holds true in this case also. At the end of the story, the starving artists have vanished, while the moralizing Maecenas occupies the stage in all his repugnant glory.

In "The Poet's Occupation" ("Het beroep van de dichter") Van Ostaijen closes in for the kill. There is no need for elaborate explanations to recognize Atupal, already familiar from "The Gang of the Trunk," as Belgium and the fictional names as flimsy disguises for contemporary writers. In this story negative aspects of the cultural world are isolated and hypertrophied.

In Atupal no one pays any attention to the work of art itself, but one judges an artist by his behavior. The critics of Atupal judge a work of art according to the degree an artist has suffered; a work of art is merely the expression of the creator and the product of his suffering. Naturally, these definitions exclude the work of art itself. In this grotesque world anti-art is the basis for the appreciation of the arts. The story's hero, the poet Jonas Baart, conforms to this absurd critical standard by writing under the name of Lachrimae Christi. Any writer of importance in Atupal has found himself similarly appropriate labels.[15]

In Atupal's literary world, literary organizations legislate taste. "Atupal has four million inhabitants and 8 million organizations. There are twice as many organizations as people. Since every organization averages 20 members, every Atupalean is a member of approximately 40 organizations. The largest number of these organizations occupy, as we are wont to call it, themselves with the cultivation of *belles-lettres*. From the conferences organized by these organizations – which are very frequent – the Atupaleans draw their literary wisdom." (III, 380) Since these organizations set the tone of literary debates concerning excellence, and since they base their judgment solely on the quantity of suffering in the artist's life, one finds here again the ever recurring principle of incorporating even such elusive matters as taste into a dictatorial force, generated by the inverse of normality. In fact, writers are forced to sham misery and deprivation in order to obtain acclaim. The story ends in an outburst of intellectual gibberish, when Lachrimae Christi tries to answer the question of why there are any poets at all in Atupal. Van Ostaijen is simply saying that there are no real poets in Atupal. They are artists by default; they have no talent to be either good waiters or good bootblacks. As can be ascertained from the other strata of this grotesque world, not one aspect of human experience is included for the right reasons. Art, too, is included for incongruous and generally selfish and utilitarian considerations. In fact, art as it is known to the normal reader does not exist in the world of the grotesque.

That Van Ostaijen was deadly serious in this attack on Belgian literary mores can be seen from a comment on this story in a speech he gave at a later date. The following passage illustrates the contention that when he satirized artistic matters, he only exaggerated what he felt to be contemporary practices.

In my sketch of their lives, I have reported rather extensively on the Atupalean poets; how, for example, in the blessed country of Atupal poems are not read at all, but how, on the contrary, the biography of even living poets is enjoyed with, I would almost say, frightening interest; furthermore, how this interest is oriented towards an exceptional interest in the trials and tribulations of the poets and how these trials and tribulations are simply identified with poetry, from which follows that the Atupalean poets, in order to please the Atupalean public are forced to organize their life in that sense, if only in appearance; from which follows that well-to-do poets find themselves forced to rent terrible garret rooms and at the same time to order, for one afternoon, a woman with a large brood which, if necessary, may consist of several broods, so that the camera man, who was commissioned by the state to film the life of Atupalean poets, can record this garret misery realistically. I do not need to add to this description the observation that the intrinsic quality of the poems has absolutely no value in Atupal. (IV, 312–313)

THE GROTESQUE AS A MORBIDLY SEXUAL UNIVERSE

One of the most persistent motifs of Van Ostaijen's grotesques is aberrant sexuality. There is hardly any story that does not have some passage describing at least one aspect of sexuality. The recurring subject of sex is but one other indication of the essential unity of Van Ostaijen's conceptual view of the world. Despite the ubiquity of sex, love or affection is, generally speaking, not very pronounced among the various manifestations of human passion. Within this world love is pathological; morbid sexuality is the norm. Selfish indulgence in hypertrophied aberrations characterizes erotic relationships. The characters are either entirely insensitive and passionless artisans of pathological love, or they fall victim to a morbid sensation of frustration. References to Freud in such tales as "Ika Loch's Brothel" and "The Gang of Trunk" indicate that this is a Freudian universe gone berserk.[16] The inmates are gathered under the banner *coito ergo sum*.

Sex and Cerebrality

Countess Angèle, the most blatant inversion of the stereotype of the young and innocent girl, lectures her decorative husband on the modality of love as pathology. During her discourse an important point is disclosed. Sex, in no matter what morbid derivation of the norm, is often represented in these tales as a cerebral phenomenon. In cases where intellect dictates sexuality, one could quite literally say that "sex is all in the mind." Angèle, for example, explains herself as a "cerebrally-sublimated hetaera." (III, 97) She is quite aware of herself as a psycho-analytic curiosity, and defends her practices clinically as being sado-masochistic. Angèle is not a person but a syndrome. Her kinetic force is reason. As she insists and demonstrates, "I went rationally towards my goal." Given her sexual deviation, she sets out to solve the problem of satisfying her sado-masochistic tendencies within the framework of social conventions. Alessandro, the truncated pseudo-Marquis de Mirlitonare, was the logical solution. Physically handicapped, he is powerless to thwart her designs, and being sexually potent, he suffers from her nightly transgressions. Every night he is put on a pedestal to watch Angèle betray him with stranger and friend alike in order to satisfy her sadism. Yet his purely decorative presence reminds her of her marital vows, hence satisfies her masochistic cravings. Indicative of grotesque justice is that the offender, Angèle, goes scot-free, while the victim, Alessandro, pays the penalty.

There is little doubt that cerebrality underlies the sexual organization of "Ika Loch's Brothel."[17] Sexual desire is based in this establishment on the madam's cerebral caprices. Ika Loch's triumph consists of turning intellectual relativity into a dictatorial tyranny, at the expense of variations of individual passions. The structure of a corporate institution, the prevalence of cerebrality in an incongruous setting and the asexuality of the madam herself combine in "Ika Loch's Brothel" to form an alien counter-image of man's sensuality. The veneer of science, of psychoanalytic knowledge and a blatantly superior attitude make Ika Loch seemingly invincible. Authority is all. Individuality, the senses, the human element are all subverted and ultimately negated. In the grotesque world one will conform or fall victim to a ruthless, impersonal force of consistent contrariness. Like Angèle, Ika Loch also ordains that sex is a physiological representation of what is essentially cerebral; i.e., anti-sexuality.

For "The General" eros is the common denominator of mankind. The General raises the erotic to a cultural standard. "But eroticism is not only sexuality; it has the overtone of human culture, of civilization in a human-biological sense. Understand from this the greater unity of people who are separated and united according to their eroticism. It is a unity on all sides." (III, 353) Pertinent to most tales is the General's notion that the erotic has aspects of both the empirical and sensual realities. The General also uses sexuality as an abstraction for his revolutionary principle of reorganizing warfare along erotic guidelines. Sexuality is an empirical and intellectual entity subject to philosophical speculation. The General joins Ika Loch and Countess Angèle in believing that there is no love but pathological love. Consequently, his model army is formed on sexual aberrations, rather than simple carnality. His plan is detailed and carefully thought out, and he assigns common sexuality a minor function in his scheme of things. Homosexuals are the elite troops; fetishists make the best artillerymen; sadists ideal shock troops; masochists the best troops for defense. (III, 354–357)

An authority on matters sexual and military, General Ricardo Gomes seems far from a healthy sexual norm himself. Theoretician *par excellence*, reality allows him only the caustic reminder of a café-owner: "The General is a pederast, but he won't show it, the dirty old man." (III, 341) The accusation of pederasty is dryly intoned again only a page later. As was the case with Ika Loch, the empirical mania for diagrammatic exposition of venereal desire is hardly based on a surfeit of personal experience. The most unqualified individuals construe the most sophisticated systems. A simple statement by the General reveals Van Ostaijen's position on a society obsessed by sex and sententious ratiocination, while its obverse characterizes the world of the grotesque. "The mind has had enough of being considered the complement of the penis." (III, 336) This sentence sums up Van Ostaijen's criticism of the world of reality. In terms of the tales it is an accurate formulation of their juxtaposing sex and ratiocination; in this world of the grotesque, the mind is indeed a complement of the genitalia.

This curious concordance between the biological and the rational urge in man has been discussed up till now from the intellectual vantage point. A slight modification in focus would indicate, however, that such a condition can easily imply its opposite, both extremes containing the same equivocation. Two traditionally opposed aspects of man's nature are conjoined as complementary reflections. Sex intellectualized or ratiocination sexualized, it is difficult indeed to ascribe hegemony to either one in this grotesque world. Libido ignites intellectual fireworks. Yet the verbal structures emasculate any potential libidinousness. One finds here one major thematic representation illustrating a negative process of this fell universe. An erosive force undermines most of organized *discordia concors*. Extremely subtle and disguised, it can only be ascertained by implication. Its result is sterile neutrality. In the present case neither the biological nor the rational urge of mankind benefits significantly from the forced conjunction. Concordance of opposites does not produce harmony, but rather an incongruity with destructive effects on both members of the equation. Any grotesque effort at unification labors towards a vacuum, towards nothingness.

Sexuality as a Force of Destruction

Sexuality as a form of absolute *verkeerdheid* has its sinister qualities too. Alessandro in "The Gang of the Trunk" is the helpless victim of Angèle's pathology. Jan Baptist Verswijfel in "Of a Windfall That Was a Misfortune" ("Van een meevallertje dat een malheur was") dies after the mysterious Ursula v. Mondschau dances naked in his club. Ursula forces members of mens' clubs to watch her peculiar performance under the threat

of armed violence: two of her impeccably dressed henchmen holding
Browning revolvers. Every time she performs someone is mesmerized by
her beauty and, unable to fulfill his longing, languishes and dies.

The hero of "The Fatal History of Scholem Weissbinder" is persecuted
by the idea of strangulation. Scholem Weissbinder is pathologically afraid
of neckties, cords and similar appendages. His preoccupation with ties in
the context of the tale might be a satire of the Freudian notion that the
necktie is a phallic symbol. The relative simplicity of his suicidal tendencies
and paranoiac delusions is infinitely complicated by eroticism. Sexually a
normal person, his desires are thwarted by feminine dress with its countless
variations of strangulation instruments. No matter how far he travels his
"invisible pursuer" follows him, and he feels that his dilemma will soon
come to a "paradoxical solution." This solution is precipitated by an erotic
adventure. On board ship he has a liaison with Dorothy, the wife of a
fellow traveller to Shanghai. The evening when Weissbinder plans to consummate his relationship with Dorothy in her cabin, the belt of her dress
throws him into paroxysms of terror. He flees, holding the belt in his hand.
"The positive desire of an affair with Dorothy turned into a negative one
for me; the notion that Dorothy, my unhappy love, was merely the external
agent of my immanent fate which, because of her, was now also becoming
erotically complicated to boot. Since that time the belt has not left me for
a moment, and I have already often been very close to strangulation." (III,
158) Weissbinder, like Telleke in "The Conviction of Notary Telleke,"
finds a paradoxical solution to his fatal persecution by the necktie (and the
belt) in committing suicide.

In "Work and Save" ("Werk en Spaar"), the inordinate passion of Breeske, a thirty-five-year-old bachelor and bank clerk, for the *demi-mondaine*
Angèle Hoedemakers, rules his life and results in nothing. Social and hier-
archical considerations are joined to the erotic theme. Breeske realizes that
his social position, particularly his lack of money, will prevent him from
ever conquering his ideal. Angèle, paradigmatic symbol of sexual beauty, is
available only to bank presidents and industrial magnates. The story, in
effect, pursues the popular notion that money buys love. Breeske systematically ruins his life to gather money. Following the principle of other
stories, he applies himself in a logical fashion to realize the slogan "work
and save." He calculates with mathematical precision how much money he
will have at a certain age, when he will still be capable of consummating
his dream. Breeske also indulges in another familiar practice in these tales;
he constantly rationalizes and demonstrates to himself the wisdom of his
actions. For example, he proves to himself that middle age, when he finally

will have saved enough money, is the best time of life to have a love affair. The narrator praises Breeske's stamina, will power, integrity – Breeske's idealism. When the day of his triumph arrives, Breeske is just in time to throw his bouquet of expensive roses on top of Angèle's casket. A basically inane little man, driven by erotic desire, is transformed into a maniacal idealist. "If one did not consider the nature of his ideal, and ideals are changing images of the times, – then Breeske had much of the integrity of Cato Uticensis. A hero of our times." (III, 168) With customary slyness, Van Ostaijen indicts the person who inspired Breeske's exemplary heroism. One of the funeral assistants dryly interrupts a woman's sentimental eulogy with the observation that if Angèle Hoedemakers had not died, she could have earned so much more money. Basically, Angèle Hoedemakers is simply a very expensive prostitute. The story assails a civilization controlled by pecuniary forces, social inequities and sexual obsessions – meager ingredients for heroic idealism.

Morbid sexuality is the foundation of a society in "The Lost House Key." Extreme preoccupation with sex drives "Camembert Or The Happy Lover" with great energy, despite the fact that he is a passionless, bourgeois little man. An aseptic stereotype of normality, he lives the unconditional worship of *das Ewig-Weibliche*. Camembert personifies normal sexuality, which is diametrically opposed to pathological love. He is, as it were, a pathological romantic. This affliction however is not preferred to Countess Angèle's fancy. Camembert's deadly immunity to passionate involvement prevents him from having opinions. Camembert is a condition: extreme bourgeois neutrality.

Camembert is completely a liaison man. The relationship leaves him cold. Not in the past. Now. The relationship is personally no longer favorable. That's why. But absolutely not cynical. Of course. If he becomes eighty, he will still be a liaison man. He won't become perverse. Sadism doesn't fit him. He is completely quietistic. Perverseness would break his quietism. That is impossible. He worships woman. He used to think that woman had to worship him. Does he still remember that? It's possible. It makes him sad. (III, 315)

"Hierarchy" bitterly burlesques the military caste system through the application of segregation by rank in a brothel. "A Marvelous Novel" verbally mocks the sultry eroticism of popular fiction and cinematography. "A History" etches the fraudulent social elite as vicious perverts. "Jus primae noctis," besides being a dialogue on Van Ostaijen's inexorable pessimism, lectures on the death of love. Love for a former mistress is delicately argued into existential listlessness, which is a reflection of the former lover's fatalistic pessimism. "Mechtildis, That Good Girl" records the philosophical musings of the stereotyped "whore with the heart of gold." "The Kiosk Girl" ("De kioskjuffrouw") is a tempered, yet wry little comment on woman's preoccupation with physical beauty. In fact, a rapid survey of Van Ostaijen's creative prose reveals that a third of the tales, including most of the longer pieces, have a pronounced preoccupation with sex. Thematically, sexuality expressed either by hyper-normality (Camembert) or hyper-aberration (Countess Angèle) is a prominent reflection of the unifying concept of a world of absolute *verkeerdheid*.

The Female as Hetaera and as Invincible Succubus

Parenthetically to this discussion of sexuality, there emerges the intriguing question of the position of women in the world of the grotesque. In "Ika Loch's Brothel" some men are negatively described as being in a succubine relationship with women. Josef la Tour, the hero of "The Kept Hotel Key," openly admits seeing woman as a succubus with Breughelian allures. Generally speaking, this is an accurate summation of the depiction of women in these tales. They have a demonic attraction and a lethal mesmeric power which draws and captures the male. Besides the suggestion of a natural force which seems to be on equal footing with the grotesque, the succubae of these tales also share, in some cases, the abusive connotation of the term. Succuba, a Late Latin form, originally meant a strumpet.[18] The combination of lasciviousness and demonic power is characteristic of a gallery of female figures in these tales. Angèle Hoedemakers ("Work and Save") is a courtesan by profession. Others are Ika Loch ("Ika Loch's Brothel") and Mechtildis ("Mechtildis, That Good Girl"). Countess Angèle should, socially and morally, also be considered a member of Mrs. Warren's profession.

Even when they are not professional hetaerae, women are hardly depicted as Victorian examples of motherhood. Adultery is quite natural in their marital relationships. The prime example is again Countess Angèle in "The Gang of the Trunk." But Dorothy, in "The Fatal History of Scholem Weissbinder," does not seem to have any compunctions either in conducting an illicit affair with a stranger. In "The Lost House Key," Paaltjes is the lover of many married women, who cherish him as an idol at the expense of their husbands. Camembert, in the story of the same name, enjoys similar favors. The red-light district figures prominently in a large number of tales: "The Gang of the Trunk," "Ika Loch's Brothel," "Human Carelessness" ("Menselijke onvoorzichtigheid"), "Camembert," "The Lost House

Key," "The Kept Hotel Key," "Hierarchy," "Mechtildis," "The General," and so on.

Such a negative appraisal of the female sex might indicate a glorification of the male. This is not the case. The male cuts a poor figure in this apparent gynaecocracy. Men usually fall victim to feminine persuasion and seduction. Ika Loch bends her male customers to her will. Countess Angèle restricts her husband to a purely decorative function, while other males are, so to speak, provisions for her pruriency. Angèle Hoedemakers in "Work and Save' is powerful enough to change a man's entire existence. Claire, in "Claire's Herd" controls the seedier elements of the town with imperial majesty. The parvenus and gay old dogs, all erotic professionals, are no match for Claire. Female superiority even assumes an archetypal stature in figures such as Promethea ("Ika Loch's Brothel"), Ursula v. Mondschau ("Of a Windfall That Was a Misfortune") and Claire ("Claire's Herd"). This female triad shares ambiguous and mystifying qualities, while their presence precipitates disaster. Claire is the most innocuous of the three, and ultimately fails to fulfill her role as demonic deity; plain normality captures her. Promethea, in "Ika Loch's Brothel," is described as a replica of the Venus Anadyomene. Despite the setting of the brothel, she impresses the reader as a deification of asexuality, as a verbalization of beauty. Yet this figure, immune to passion and depicted as sterilized beauty, triggers and falls herself victim to a mysterious murder which, paradoxically, seals the success of Ika Loch's curious establishment. Her mere presence precipitates violence.

Ursula v. Mondschau ("Of a Windfall That Was a Misfortune") is, of the three, perhaps the most fitting symbol of the succubus. She is described with verbal nuances, rather than with bold fictional strokes, in a manner analogous to Promethea.[19] Like Promethea, her appearance leads to inevitable disaster. Ursula appears to meetings of mens' clubs without having been invited. While two men in her employ hold the members at gunpoint, Ursula performs an exotic dance in the nude, and disappears just as suddenly as she came. Her beauty, like Promethea's, is almost beyond belief. Her dance is described as non-erotic. Yet her appearance draws men like Jan Baptist Verswijfel, and makes them look for her until their fruitless search ends in death. Unfulfilled longing for this paradigmatic apparition kills them. Ursula is not innocent of these strange deaths: she has a filing-system with a large number of cards recording the names and death notices of many men. Like a true demonic spirit, she kills men with her beauty. The motive? Van Ostaijen provides the following ambiguous explanation. Ursula is the most perfect of female beauties. Her beauty is so superior that she herself is, as it were, abstractly in love with herself. She is disappointed in the male veneration which she feels is her due. It is not commensurate with her surpassing beauty. This disappointment leads her to venerate herself. The latter thought is expressed in her dance. "A moral dance from the severe period of the Lycurgan cult of the body." (III, 150) One of the armed gentlemen who accompany her on her escapades carefully argues a defense of Ursula's activities. It is the combination of the appearance of Ursula and the peculiar defense which induces men like Verswijfel to look for her, firm in their conviction that they are the expression of the humble veneration demanded by Ursula.

These enigmatic figures have elicited little response from critics. Yet their ambiguous presence warrants an explanation which they seem diligently to avoid. The preponderance of the erotic in these tales requires a discussion which, in turn, inevitably leads to probing these statuesque figures. Within the context of the grotesque world, they appear to occupy an antithetical position to a morbid and diseased society. Succubae are an irrational rebuttal of a grotesque and tainted world. The women associated with this idea (Angèle, Ursula, Promethea, Claire) are immune to nefarious consequences of the grotesque. They victimize, but are never victims. For even when death cuts short their fictional existence, as in the case of Promethea, it does not alter them measurably, but instead seems to enforce their suprahuman existence. The choice of succubae was a happy one. Their irrational powers and mystery immunize them against the grotesque. Their purported lasciviousness fits the world in which they appear.

In a world of unlimited license, these females exercise a hold which no one can resist. Paradigmatic outlaws, they remain unassailed by the incongruous congruity of the grotesque. Being essentially axiomatic derivations from the norm, they need not be distorted by the grotesque's lens. These figures legislate a strange justice. Ursula, a paradigm of beauty, chastises an insufficient veneration of herself as an ideal. Angèle eradicates the sanctity of matrimony which has become insolvent under bourgeois management, and deifies lawless love. Claire personifies archetypal femininity or atavistic sensuality, and remains unmolested in the refined lubricious society of *rastas* and *vieux-marcheurs*. Promethea casts a spell of beauty which hypnotizes even the most stolid of Ika Loch's clientele. Their common denominator is beauty. While they emit a perilous fascination, they are not pure ideality. Yet the sinister alloy of these figures is all the more effective. Decorative emblems of tainted beauty, they are perhaps the only representation of an ideal order in this world of the grotesque. It is all the more fitting that their sublimity is tarnished, since the grotesque has no place for a Pantheon.

The only male figures who enjoy a similar immunity from grotesque repurcussions are Wybau ("Patriotism Incorporated") and Knackfuss ("The Gang of the Trunk"). They are the fuglemen of the grotesque. In both cases, Van Ostaijen carefully documents their exotic (i.e., anti-bourgeois) origins. Both have commonplace fathers, but exotic mothers. Both are exponents of a pessimistic neutrality, which allows them to practice any vice of the grotesque world without being tainted or corrupted. Wybau and Knackfuss are so consistently unethical and amoral, that they are superior to any fraudulence any grotesque character might contemplate. Both are epitomes of the outlaw. In the world of license, the outlaw is king.

A GROTESQUE DEMOCRACY

Almost all of Van Ostaijen's protagonists are abstractions of various aspects of the grotesque. Negative uniformity accentuates the unity of the tales, while at the same time demonstrating the theoretical prognostications of the Breughel-essay. Emphasis is on extraneous creation. The artist maintains distance from his work, maintains creative neutrality. *Schöpferische Indifferenz* is hardly a good recipe for dramatic characterization. The inhabitants of this fictional world are the puppets Van Ostaijen mentioned in his essay – puppets set into motion by remote control. The source of control is folly. Similarity is again emphasized by their identical speech. Quite literally, they are animated figures of speech. The characters of the grotesque world are mostly mere tropes of folly. Any juxtaposition of a speech fragment in one tale with one from another will corroborate this statement. The General's argument for prototypal warfare is no different from Angèle's argumentative discourse on her sado-masochistic behavior. Everything in these tales aids in depicting the essential, basic unity of absolute *verkeerdheid*. The adjective *absolute* insists on the abstraction of the fundamental idea. Unity of theme calls for unity of tone. In all of the longer tales one finds the incongruous erudition of the characters. From the point of view of rhetoric, the politicians of "Patriotism Incorporated" have no verbal edge on the Berlin prostitute Mechtildis. As usual, the expected does not materialize. One simply does not anticipate a streetwalker sounding like a professor of metaphysics.

There is in most tales a thematic parataxis. The "superior" strata of society are very often equated or set side by side with the lowest ones. In "The Gang of the Trunk" there is an exact reversal when the gang, lead by

Knackfuss, assimilates with nobility without very much difficulty. Alessandro, it may be remembered, is almost like the twin of the noble Marquis de Mirlitonare. A Peruvian General holds court in the dives of Antwerp's waterfront. Intricate intellectual curlicues adorn the conversation in Ika Loch's brothel. In the "Intermezzo" of the metaphysical theatre, scholars and authors rub shoulders with journeymen. Syphilis creates a culture in "The Lost House Key." The film scenario "Bankruptcy Jazz" unites seamstress and members of parliament under the auspices of jazz and inflation. This "democracy" of the tales is summed up in "Claire's Herd"; "between Claire and Christ there is only the difference in the degree of their respective concentration." (III, 307) Van Ostaijen's depiction of the seamier side of the city has a matter-of-factness about it, as if it were the most logical background for seasoned and eloquent speakers.[20] Reiteration, similarity of tone and theme, unity of style and outlook combine to form a phylogenetic, rather than an ontogenetic interpretation of fictional characters.

Thematic parataxis produces a presentiment of alienation and estrangement. Distortion by hypertrophy or atrophy is the essential earmark of these grotesques. Juxtaposing contemplative cerebrality and a harbor's red-light district invokes a shudder of apprehension. Concomitant with apprehensive presentiment, this procedure clears the way for abstraction. What's expected fictionally does not happen and is in conflict with the massive architectonics of language. The result of this conflict is increasing abstraction. The construction of these tales aids in eliciting fear in the reader. Having read the first sentence or paragraph, the reader has ambled into a *cul de sac*. There is no way out. He must follow the relentless inevitability of the grotesque's mathematical progression, which parodies certainty. A negligible factor grows into a national, global or cosmic presence. Losing a house key is the foundation of a civilization ("The Lost House Key"); an advertising slogan controls a man's life ("Work and Save"). This ex-centric movement corresponds to the demonic inevitability of *verkeerdheid*. In the following passage Van Ostaijen sums up the stylistic principle and its thematic counterpart in a very apt comparison.

A stone which falls into the water makes first a small circle. In an instant the circle has enlarged itself into ten, twenty circles, which gradually grow wider up to the very edges of the water. Social life in the city is like this. The larger circle issues spontaneously and biologically-necessary from the second. The stone moves the entire city. The outer edges know nothing of the initial action. They only know that they vibrated a larger circle because the previous circle was larger again than the one that preceded it. (III, 308)

It is quite obvious that this is applicable to the losing of the house key in "The Lost House Key," building in "City of Builders," Ika Loch's fame in "Ika Loch's Brothel," the brothel in "Hierarchy," and so on.

The application of this principle gives the illusion of wandering through a maze or labyrinth. One has the illusion of being guided with assurance. At the end of the fictional adventure assurance turns into a shudder of horror, uncomfortable laughter, or a sense of being left alone in threatening darkness. Van Ostaijen provided an apt metaphor. In two prominent places he makes use of the myth of Ariadne and Theseus. The clew of thread which she gave to the Greek hero, and which lead him out of the labyrinth after having killed the Minotaur, this clew of Ariadne is the title of one of the collections of prose pieces. But in the story "The Fatal History of Scholem Weissbinder," there is a passage which describes the negative sense of being led through a maze by danger, and not towards deliverance.

The more I attempt to flee the calamity, the more certain it is that I am going towards it. Each step brings me deeper into Minos' dangerous labyrinth. And I don't even have the hope of being rescued by Ariadne's clew of thread. No, all aid, every relaxation with a distracting pleasure casts me deeper into misfortune. This is what the thread of Ariadne must be to me, unless I cannot conquer the inclination to regard it as rope, so that, instead of showing me the way out of the horrible labyrinth of my torment, it only becomes an object which pursues me in its turn. (III, 157)

Cul de sac, concentric circles, labyrinth, Ariadne's thread which strangles instead of liberates – all these overlapping notions stress the grotesque's omnipotent absurdity and the relentless and cathegorical pursuit of *verkeerdheid*. In this conspiratorial universe, the reader's credulity is undermined. Having been lured into the game of the grotesque, the reader finds himself odd man out.

Having emphasized the malevolent nature of the grotesque, one might be puzzled by the ubiquity of the characters' consistent idealism. H. Uyttersprot was the first to isolate this incongruous preoccupation of the characters in his incisive essay *Paul van Ostaijen and his prose*. Most of the characters are radical logicians of a perverse idealism. Pameelke's superpatriotism becomes an idealistic absurdity vigorously defended by Wybau, the totally noncommitted man. Angèle propounds a theory in support of her own idealistic self-conception as a "cerebrally sublimated hetaera." Ika Loch doggedly pursues the ideal of a brothel based on scientific principles. Prisoner No. 200 follows his will-to-prison in an exemplary fashion. The municipal authorities of Creixcroll turn into fanatical builders. General Ricardo Gomes holds a logical discourse on pure martiality. Mechtildis, the

Berlin streetwalker, defends her occupation as purely idealistic philanthropy. Examples are plentiful. All these scholastics of the incongruous are radical idealists. Throughout the tales the lengthy ratiocinations share clusters of recurring terms: idealist, idealism, mania, unconditional, will-to-something, absolute, must, etc. However, one should not be misled by the urgency and brilliant subtlety of their arguments. For one thing, these tales could be seen as a plea for a reality beyond the madness of the grotesque universe. Familiarity with the entirety of Van Ostaijen's work might lead to such a positive conclusion. But within the context of the groesques, it is yet another reflection of a single purpose. Van Ostaijen depicts a world of absolute *verkeerdheid*. The adjective *absolute* provides one clue for the epistemological argumentation. The tales are rational apostrophes of axiomatic incongruity; apostrophes of ideal counterfeiting, ideal infidelity, ideal martiality, ideal prostitution, ideal chauvinism, ideal building, and so on. Each of these tales is faithful to the central preoccupation – presenting an absolute of folly. With an entire battery of philosophical, verbal and rational devices, these characters attempt to persuade us of the sublimity of their insidious world.

Like an abstract *circulus in probando* the tales, more often than not, end in silence or the absurd. Ika Loch's desire for a scientific brothel is the cause of her success, while it shows her, at the same time, as incapable of such a venture. No. 200 obtains his prison in heaven, not knowing that it is a metaphysical fraud. The General's seminar on pure warfare is subverted by the infamous setting of Antwerp's waterfront and his casually mentioned suicide. Breeske's rational monologues and heroic pursuit of the ideal are negated by the death of the *demi-mondaine*. Of course, from the characters' point of view, their fantastic ratiocinations are perfectly rational and plausible. They feel that they are quite practical in their Socratic pursuit of self-knowledge. Even the hypertrophy of style strives for total inclusiveness, which merely counterpoints the pandemic grotesque universe of the tales.

The significance of these idealistic discourses seems to be threefold. First of all, this mode of cerebral exposition argues essential incongruity to its preordained absurd absolute. In so doing it tries to trap the reader into believing its arguments by the sheer weight of erudition. Its method is essentially inductive, and parallels Van Ostaijen's overriding desire to depict a universe of catholic grotesqueness. Finally, this clausal mode of discursive writing, as opposed to the dramatic or narrative mode, enhances the impression of abstraction. Thematically, Van Ostaijen plays with and parodies man's overconfidence in his verbal and rational superstructures. As these tales prove, a different focusing produces an entirely different effect from what is expected. A slight deviation from the norm presents an antithetical modality which – in its consistent relativism – has equal right to our attention. Like many other artistic modes, these tales develop an oblique premise logically. Such oblique focusing presents a prostitute who defends her occupation as being idealistic and philanthropic. Nevertheless, it remains absurd to meet a philosopher-whore, especially one who proves herself to be an ardent logician.

A GROTESQUE WITH A DIFFERENCE: THE REBELLION OF JOSEF LA TOUR

Everything in the foregoing discussion stressed the autonomy of the dictatorial grotesque. The characters are perfectly adjusted to this upside-down world, and never question its validity. Indeed they demonstrate against normality, and their intense demonstrations mark them as fanatical apologists of the grotesque. For our sober intellects, presumably geared to healthy normal standards, their most unnerving quality is their unawareness of abnormal behavior, fallacious reasoning, their world of Folly Incorporated. The characters file past like a set of palimpsests. Their similarity, despite the most outrageous situations, only reinforces the permeating strength of the grotesque. They seem never to question the order in which they live, or attempt to be disloyal to it. As abstractions they are most congenial to the grotesque organism. What would happen if such a character would suddenly be infected by doubt? Is there such a character, and is there a tale in which such a character is the hero? If so, would there be any modifications of the grotesque norm just described?

The tale which answers positively to these rhetorical questions is "The Kept Hotel Key." Its hero and his millieu is Van Ostaijen's arch-enemy, the bourgeois. Other major elements of the grotesque can be found in the story. But its major point of interest is its hero, Josef la Tour, who tries to break through the grotesque into an ambivalent ideality. La Tour is the missing link between the world of our experience and the world of the grotesque. Being closer (to whatever degree this may be) to our normal sphere of reference, he is more dramatically realized than the other characters. He does not indulge in pyramidal logical demonstrations; he is more realistically drawn. In short he is more human. Van Ostaijen pits this understudy of humanity against the grotesque universe. Josef la Tour is a bourgeois by his own admission. Van Ostaijen even allows him to present a backhanded compliment to his breed. The middle-class' inevitably negative capability is found to have at least one positive function.

I say that the burgher has many good qualities. I could prove to you that, if art still exists, we have to thank the burgher for it. The burgher rejects all art. This is a great service, however, because at the same time, he breaks the necks of all dilettantes. Ultimately, one can reject only what is rejectable. I see the burgher as a kind of security police for art. His work is negative only. Without that negative quality, we cannot progress. ((III, 361)

On the surface La Tour seems a normal middle-class man with a simplistic sense of epicurism: "a good glass of beer, sometimes a shot of brandy, a glass of port in the morning a good-looking woman in bed, and there you have my philosophy of the joy of life." He is a fairly well-educated man, who is conventionally married. His wife is devoted to him, while he leads the normal double life of husband and *bon vivant*. The wife is a good sort who rather sees him drinking than running after women. She is absolutely convinced of his fidelity.

However, it soon becomes clear that La Tour is not the Telleke type; he is a burgher with a difference. Within the context of the grotesque world he has one lethal flaw: awareness, awareness of himself and the insuffiency of his existence. In a series of negative polarities, Van Ostaijen records obliquely the widening rift between La Tour and his world. The story is an elaborate Kierkegaardian dilemma without the "leap of faith." Other characters do not question the absurdity of their mania. Their absolute conviction of its normality provides them with inexhaustible energy. But La Tour questions; La Tour doubts. This *rara avis* chooses disquiet and anxiety in this efficiently run grotesque aviary. La Tour describes himself as an intermediary between a caricature of Molière and a "victim of black magic." He freely confesses to his succubine relationship with women. His succubus is not intellectualized, he insists, not a "cognac-and-coffee-whore," but an atavistic creature from the world of Breughel. In fact, he is haunted by the spectre of absolute *verkeerdheid*.

La Tour is, to a degree, a split personality: a bourgeois and a mystic. The incommensurability between these two extreme polarities dooms him, but does not prevent him from seeking a metaphysical solution. La Tour revolts against vulgar mediocrity. His revolt takes the form of a concurrent desire for two absolutes, absolute sublimity and absolute evil. He has, he says, one foot in Jerusalem and one in Babel. Incapable of living a normal life, he constantly pursues extremes while at the same time trying to extricate himself from this battle of contrasts. Absolute evil, logically enough, has strong sexual overtones. A man not content with vulgar mediocrity, La Tour searches for his atavistic succubus. He searches for her in the lowliest levels of society and fails to find her. The lethal attraction of the grotesque, personified by La Tour's chimera of a demonic absolute of erotic vulgarity, forces him to haunt Brussels' most degenerate establishments. At this point La Tour's demise begins. To his horror he suddenly realizes, amidst the prostitutes, pimps, and other professionals of vice, that they are merely vulgar. In one of Van Ostaijen's most bitter passages comes the discovery that the illusion of total depravity, which may be assumed to flourish in this milieu, is but conventional.

> This whore was the most middle class tea-time. Whores, pimps, and clientele played with each other in a jovial convention. The boss was the most active in this convention. People understood each other marvelously. The women stank of bourgeoisie. He conjured up for himself the most stupid illusions. That these women would have an idea of the demonic. He crawled for a woman, and she became afraid of his crawling. The height of her demonism was to get into bed and collect 100 francs. (III, 366–7)

La Tour discovers that the demonic is not an aspect of the grotesque. Despite its sinister and insidious character, the grotesque is basically conventional. The implications are subtle, but devastating. Van Ostaijen has dealt the final blow; he has negativised negativity. There is a subtle horror in this ultimate explanation of absolute *verkeerdheid*. It would have been more understandable or acceptable to find the grotesque in the shape of Beelzebub, in the shape of something larger than life. That way it would gain stature, become a worthy opponent, allow one to draw clear lines of battle. The pessimism is all the more devastating upon finding that the grotesque's great strength lies in the anonymity of incarnate mediocrity; the bourgeoisie. Like a medieval zealot, La Tour frantically tries to wrench absolute evil from conventional degeneracy. He yearns to be broken, to be eradicated by a force larger than life. But monolithic normality frustrates his most desperate attempts. Impotence and frustration seethe in this tale as in no other. Van Ostaijen has to some degree trangressed the rule of neutrality and objectivity laid down in the Breughel essay. The artist has allowed himself proximity to his subject. Involvement demands the price of suffering. Intense frustration betrays itself in a barely controlled hatred.

Not only absolute evil, but also sublimity is neutralized by mediocrity. Josef tries to force desperate perversities on the prostitutes he encounters. His eroticism expresses itself in hatred and even in physical violence. But no matter how low he stoops, hoping to attain (quite literally) abnormality, he is constantly rebuffed by stolid conventionality. For example, the mercantile code of the prostitutes prescribes that payment allows perversities; his most violent and perverse actions therefore are condoned and thereby neutralized. Evil is also neutralized when La Tour discovers whores having the saintly faces of portraits by Van Eyck. "He took a woman and begged, be unfaithful to me. She put her Madonna head in his lap." [21] In "The Kept Hotel Key" sex has finally been sterilized completely. Ika Loch set the stage with her aseptic brothel. Countess Angèle normalized pathological love. Now the world of vice and sexual abnormality has become as pedestrian as daily reality. "Life was a dog's life; Josef couldn't stand the sight of another beer. Activity in the city was tame. The trams clanged incessantly, that was all." (III, 369) The contrast Madonna/prostitute or Jerusalem/Babel is a lie. La Tour finds a conclusion which, at least, cancels the polarities; "Life was the most common banality." [22]

At that moment a new contrast, a more venomous one, disturbs the resignation of total pessimism. Bourgeois morality, embodied by his wife, stirs guilt in his soul. Her implacable innocence and doglike devotion nauseate him and, at the same time, castigate his conscience. Josef admits to himself that he hates her too. She persecutes him with tenderness. Having discovered a measure of peace through total abjection and immense pessimism, a negative peace, which could allow him a respite of some sort, he must now start all anew to purge this subtler monster from his life. Here it is relevant to quote once more the passage on pessimism from "Jus primae noctis," which so accurately describes Van Ostaijen's position.

Pessimism in itself as a philosophy would be deliverance for me. And a great wealth. That I can not have. Everything has become flat with me because I did not desire the abstract consistently. Consider this pessimism with comparisons oriented toward the outside world. Everything is such a pitiful mess. (III, 13)

The last sentence echoes Josef's "life is a dog's life." The only difference between this passage and Josef's bitter discovery is that he did, indeed, "desire the abstract consistently." But the longing found no fulfillment, and banal neutrality is condemning him to death. Now he hates his wife Marianne with a vehemency equal to that with which he hated the prostitutes. The one shows him the vulgarity of banality, the other the banality of vulgarity. Disgusted and defeated, he returns home. But with him goes an objective correlative of his defeat, of his remorse, of his guilt, of his desire for release.

In his pocket he discovers a hotel key which he forgot to return after his last, violent dèbâcle with the young prostitute Angèle. Though he reminds himself repeatedly that he will send it back, Josef knows full well he will never do so. The key is a symbol of the constant negation of himself. Josef tries to tell his wife the truth, but her innocent docility and painful vulnerability frighten him into silence and lies. At one point he even indulges in a bit of familiar ratiocination about his guilt, about the key and the duality of body and soul, Babel and Jerusalem. But it is an intellectual ruse. The truth of the dilemma he presents in less stylized utterings. In a jumble of halftruths and peripheral observations, one line of thought begins to develop. Josef continues to detest conventional mediocrity. He would like to destroy the serene happiness of his wife. What prevents him is partly his guilt, but, more importantly, the thought that she would not hate him, that after this death she would become merely indifferent to his former existence.

Josef still yearns for a *Steigerung* of existence, and continues to abhor neutrality and indifference. He confesses to the narrator that he desires to leave life, but that he cannot do so as long as someone loves him. However, the one who does so is Marianne, and her placid, grey quotidian variety is not sufficiently abnormal or absolute to kill himself for. Guilt is prominent in his mind, but he admits that he is not quite sure what he is guilty about. His hatred spurs him on to deny love vehemently. The bitter irony of his life is that the only true love he knows is of the wrong kind. Finally, he does tell Marianne of his sins, adding, however, that he is not quite himself any longer. Marianne is concerned and anxious about his illness. Josef has been foiled once more.

In "Jus primae noctis" Van Ostaijen states that suicide is either "an unconquered point of view or a relapse into infantilism. The only attainable happiness is to know the incurable misery of life." (III, 10) Telleke and Weissbinder commit suicide to prevent an absurdity; in a sense their demise is a relapse into infantility. General Ricardo Gomes also commits suicide. His death is somewhat ludicrous, when seen in relation to his inspired martiality. Josef la Tour commits suicide out of frustration, from the realization of "an unconquered point of view." He has obviously not attained the resigned pessimism of finding a measure of contentment in the incurability of life's misère. Even in the final hours of his life, on the quays of Antwerp's waterfront, frustration and harsh indifference persecute him. While he is trying to drink some courage into himself, a barmaid thinks he is going "to pull a heist," and asks him to buy her some underwear. Vulgar banality and mediocrity will not release their hold over him. "There is really not much space on the docks. Not even there." The death of Josef la Tour is a final desperate gesture of defeat. Grotesque mediocrity has conquered.

Some attention was concentrated on this story since it presents a counterpoint to the other major grotesques. Familiar themes of the bourgeois and sexuality form the background of the tale. In "The Kept Hotel Key" sexuality's morbidity is cauterized. The Freudian universe of pathological love is reduced to the triviality of a lady's club. The erotic is vulgar banality. Impermeable mediocrity never quite attained the sinister supremacy it does in "The Kept Hotel Key." This tale graphically, and in a manner less para-

bolic than in some of the others, illustrates Von Ostaijen's "bitter knowledge of human actions." (IV, 278) Inutility of action precipitates Josef la
Tour's suicide. An undertow of violence lurks beneath the story's main
stream of frustration. In it one finds also a formulation of the polarity Van
Ostaijen speaks of in his Breughel essay. Josef la Tour reaches for both
Jerusalem and Babel. Relinquishing the former, he feels that at least
paradigmatic evil should be within his grasp. But the incommensurability
between ordinary existence and an ideal, even a negative absolute, only
widens the chasm of nil. Death finally promises the only release from
frustation.

Why does this particular story seem a more intimate disclosure of Van
Ostaijen's central preoccupations? The answer lies in the narrative presentation. Josef la Tour is not one of the human marionettes who dance their
stately antic in the other major grotesques. Van Ostaijen has not adhered
to the consistent objectivity noted in the other tales. The *Verfremdungseffekt*, more residual in this story, is contained in the relationship between
Josef la Tour and his fictional universe; that is to say, it develops organically
from within the story. In the other tales, it does not evolve from within the
story, but from the confrontation between its absolute incongruity and the
reader's preconceptions of congruity. "The Kept Hotel Key" is dramatic
narrative. For once Van Ostaijen betrayed his mode of strict objectivity.
The aesthetic detachment of the other grotesques has made way for a more
emotional awareness of tragedy. Always the conscientious artist, Van Ostaijen differentiates this tale from his other stories. "The Kept Hotel Key"
is designated as a tragicomedy, a "grotesque with a tear." "It became a
grotesque with a tear, and it had, at the same time, a ridiculous tragic
character." (III, 369) At one point Josef sees his life as a "sad comedy"
and Van Ostaijen, the narrator, calls it with frustrated sympathy a "ridiculous history."

The story shows that emotional awareness and a sense of the tragic are
not indigenous to the gelid severity of the grotesque's unmitigated incongruity. In the other tale of a key ("The Lost House Key"), Hasdrubal
Paaltjes played his mechanical role as the Adam of a brave new syphilitic
world. Josef la Tour, conscious of his humanity and striving to break
through the sinister banality of the grotesque, discovered himself straddling
a meaningless vacuum. La Tour was forced to execute himself because he
lived a fictional life at a disadvantage. He did not play the game of the
grotesque according to its rules. Playing metaphysical poker with the grotesque is like playing with loaded dice against a computer. Feelings are
detrimental. Humanity is the loser, and must pay the heavy price of extinction.

VAN OSTAIJEN AND MYNONA:
"LUDIC" ART VERSUS SOCIAL SOLEMNITY

As a postcript to these pages, a final note on the playful side of Van Ostaijen's art. Here he has something in common with a little known German writer of "Grotesken," Mynona, pseudonym for Salomon Friedlaender (1871–1946). Fairly recent epistolary discoveries have revealed that Van Ostaijen was well acquainted with him, and his occasional allusions to Mynona's work in his essays and tales show that he had also read Mynona't works. To clarify Van Ostaijen's brand of humor, a descriptive parallel with Mynona's theories of the comic, particularly in his *Unroman, Die Bank der Spötter* (München, 1919), might be instructive. The type of humor of both these writers is intellectual and sophisticated. Merciless, strident, their humor exposes what is conceived as the organic disease of human life. This humor is militant as well as cerebral. "Erst eine wütende Idee ist Idee . . . Exploitieren wir die Kanaille der Idee, die Menschheit, bis sie begreifen lernt." (*Bank*, 259) Mynona, perhaps the most subtle and refined intellectual humorist of modern German literature did, like his Flemish acquaintance, recognize the power of nuances. Not only broad humor, but also sly pinpricks can have the same desired effect of eliciting a reaction from its human target. The first has the immediate impact which might conveniently be forgotten, while the other works on the principle of delayed reaction. "Man wirft nicht nur Bomben des Humors . . . man schleudert auch leichte, kitzelnde Lanzen, kämpft mit allen Waffen, nicht nur mit schweren Geschütz. Ich traume immer, es gebe einen ganz feinen Punkt; wer diesen träfe . . . der müsste einen solchen Lacherfolg haben, dass noch der Tod selber sich lebendig lachte anstatt dass jetzt die meisten lachenden Leute sich zu Tode lachen." (*Bank*, 383) If Van Ostaijen thought of objectivity as the indirection of Breughel's humor, Mynona writes of a similar mode, which does not loudly proclaim humor's adversary, but rather one "welche sich freilich verschweigt, verstellt und statt ihrer direkten Offenbarung nur das Verlachte zum Vorschein bringt." (*Bank*, 40)

In the case of Van Ostaijen, the direct representation would be absolute *verkeerdheid*, but he chooses the indirect method of presenting "das Verlachte" in a series of grotesque topoi such as inflation, counterfeiting, patriotism, pathological sexuality, etc. What, on the surface, might appear as a playing with form and the satiric mode hides a very serious intention of the author, only revealed through the proces of indirect communication. Mynona insists on a similar profundity in his verbal antics. "Beachten Sie nur die Kontraste zwischen kindischem Spiel und hohem Sinn! Der Menschheit ganzer Jammer klagt heimlich-unheimlich in dieser scheinbaren Hans-wurstiade." (*Bank*, 44) In a passage from his "anti-novel," Mynona provides an incisive formulation of his own goals, and moreover, summarizes the intended impact as well as content of Van Ostaijen's grotesques.

Quichote kämpfte gegen Windmühlen, weil er sie für starke Feinde hielt. Er halluzinierte heroische Gefahren, wo die Banalität des Alltags existierte. Für uns aber sind die ernsthaftesten Wirklichkeiten nur Windmühlen, nicht war? Was bedeutet für uns z.B. ein Staat? Ein Blindenheim? Ein Feldherr? Oder glauben Sie, dass uns etwa ein Fürstenhof hoheren Respekt abnötigen würde? Glauben Sie das tatsächlich? Sie wissen, dass alle diese durchaus nicht nur eingebildeten Veranstaltungen, diese Militarismen, Ministerien, Parlamente, Börsen, Trusts, Theater, alle diese Menschen, Tiere, Sachen, Sonnen, Kometen und Planeten für unsereinen nur willkommenen Anlass zum Spott angeben. Bewahre! Unser Idea-lismus ist sehend, nicht blind wie der des Quichote. (*Bank*, 257)
Wir hier sind desillusionierte Quichotes: wir sehen nicht nur Windmühlen, sehen unsere Dulcinea nicht nur als viehdumme Magd, welche noch dazu untreu ist; sondern die ganze Menschenwelt von ihren Sternen an bis zu ihren Läusen und noch tiefer hinab, nicht wahr, finden wir realiter beherrscht von Irrtum, Wahnwitz, Verzerrung und Verderben. Aber nicht wie Hamlet, bitte, wollen wir darüber weinen. Wir sind die Lachenden. Die Liebhaber der Idee . . . (*Bank*, 258)

Certainly anyone acquainted with Van Ostaijen's grotesques will see the striking similarities between Mynona's description of his *Hanswurstiade* and Van Ostaijen's world of absolute *verkeerdheid*. Notice the similar dis-like of social institutions such as the military (Van Ostaijen's "The General" and "Hierarchy"), governmental departments ("Patriotism Incorporated" and "The Prison in Heaven"), parliaments ("Patriotism Incorporated"), national economies ("The Adventures of Mercurius"), and corporate insti-tutions ("Patriotism Incorporated"). Van Ostaijen rallied to Mynona's battlecry: "Aus der Freiheit der Gedanken in die Schranken der Sinnenwelt als Missionare der Idee einbrechen! Nicht der Idealismus, sondern dessen Feigheit vor der Realität ist abgetan; das verkennen diese realistisch-posi-tivistischen Damen." (*Bank*, 384)

But at this juncture Mynona and Van Ostaijen part ways. Van Ostaijen is not like Mynona's "lachende Idealist," who sees the world existing thanks to a "sich selber immerfort kitzelnden Schöpfer." Mynona the writer of gro-tesques and his alter-ego, Salomon Friedlaender the Kantian, share a cosmic optimism, which not even the *Irrtum* of reality could destroy. Mynona's peculiar philosophy of radiant cosmosophy, grounded on Kant and Ernst Marcus, is a mystico-cerebral galaxy far removed from Van Ostaijen's conditional futility. Not even a laborious exposition proving a tenuous positivism for Van Ostaijen's lyricism, his professed joy in the creative act, the harmony of the self-sustaining work of art, none of these could possibly resemble Mynona's sweeping thought of cosmic celebration as it is displayed in his "anti-novels" *Die Bank der Spötter* and *Der Schöpfer*. Such a conception is far removed from Van Ostaijen's weary resignation, as it is formulated in a letter to the Dutch writer and friend E. du Perron. "A book counts only for the small piece of truth which it reveals. *Hamlet* is one of the greatest creations because there the small piece of truth is bigger than elsewhere. (The truth of the inevitability of man's ultimate defeat.)" [23] But short of Mynona's final telescopic vision, his and Van Ostaijen's purpose and practice of the comic mode, of literary, cerebral humor, are very close indeed.

Despite the gravity of the tales' intentions, one must never lose sight of the playful, the capricious side of Van Ostaijen's art. When the act of creation is a positive action, is an intellectual and spiritual joy, there must be a lighter vein which runs both counter to and parallel with the themes in a minor key. These intricate arabesques of the grotesque world are intellectual *concetti*, which almost seem to taunt the stolid negativity of the world of absolute *verkeerdheid*. Van Ostaijen became never accustomed to the overbearing seriousness of much of Dutch and Flemish literature at the time. One spoke of the vicissitudes of life in large, expansive gestures of a grave and responsible person. No matter how serious a Fool might be in his tragicomic antics, he is anathema to the decent middle-class man. Van Ostaijen wanted to set poetry free from the stifling atmosphere of weighty respectability.

In a review of new work by six Dutch poets, Van Ostaijen airs his dislike of what became almost synonymous with the Dutch nation: *plechtigheid*. *Plechtigheid* combines "solemnity," "ceremoniousness," being "dignified," "stately," and "imposing"; it excludes a sense of humor, especially where it concerns one's own personage. This "solemnity-mentality" ("plechtigheidsmentaliteit") must be reflected in imposing verse which prevents, according to Van Ostaijen, a centripetal force of words in isolation; "the solemn formulation grows like fungus, only in width." (IV, 158) He calls his own work "non-serious lyricism," and proposes that one should outlaw for "35 years" the word "serious" in Holland, as well as slapping a heavy fine on the use of the word *dignified*. He characterizes the solemnity of the Lowlands, which includes Flanders, with this sarcastic observation about Holland's fate. "But it is – I say, perhaps – as long as there's life there's hope – but it is, or better, it appears to be the fate of the Lowlands by the sea that the inhabitants do not know what to do with seriousness and that ministers function there at the same time as directors of the circus. That's a pity. Because a circus is a beautiful thing as long as no minister is its director." (IV, 315)

To show how emancipated the Dutch have become in the intervening years, consider the following appreciation of Van Ostaijen's prose by A. H. Gomperts in his excellent essay on the Flemish writer.[24]

The playful, satirical writings of Paul van Ostaijen are in contrast to the weightiness of the publication a constant assault on Seriousness, fat, weighty Seriousness, which he found to be particularly characteristic of Northern Dutch literature. This opinion is partly to blame for his limited fame. He was too playful for our seriousness and too intellectual for the kind of stupid festiveness which was so popular in Flanders. Paul van Ostaijen was, therefore, a writer who fell between chairs. He has just received some new attention, because the poets who appeared after the Second World War recognized in his poetic experiments, which grew out of the climate of the First World War, a kindred spirit and a precursor.

Once the lyric was given a new lease on life as an autonomous organism outside all other, non-lyrical considerations, it could as easily juggle fire as well as waterballs. "Summing-up I say, the poem, just like conjuring, is its own end. A noticeable difference between these two does not exist. Only that the poem is the conjuring of the poet. There is, therefore, a difference of level. While conjuring does not carry its own explanation along with it, the poem-conjuring trick contains an *a priori* point of view beyond conjuring: a way in which to conceive of things, indeed a way to conceive of phenomena." (IV, 115) Naturally, this theory of poetry is a reflection of Van Ostaijen's basic dislike of the bourgeois. For the burgher, poetry must be serious, otherwise it has not enough weight to convince him of its importance. It is plain effrontery to declare that poetry is a game of words. "With the wooden blocks of my set, I make now a church, now a house, sometimes even something which is neither church nor house, only the desire to put the blocks on top of each other. Someone says that this is not playing according to the rules of art; you must stick to the model. And my friend who thinks his homework a game, calls my game decadence." (IV, 116)

Most of his essays on literature are a joust with the powerful Flemish literary establishment, which considered Van Ostaijen's strident and impertinent utterances about the lightness of the lyric a slap in the face of Art. They would not stand for Terpsichore pinching Melpomene. Nor could they fathom the seriousness of Van Ostaijen's *ludic* theories of poetry, the profundity of his light, but serious lyrical game, implied in his famous statement: "Poetry is not: thought, spirit, well-turned phrases, neither doctoral nor dada. It is simply a game of words anchored in the meta-physical." (IV, 380)

It is therefore not surprising that in the grotesques he delighted in taking such subjects under scrutiny as patriotism ("Patriotism Incorporated"), prostitution ("Ika Loch's Brothel"), counterfeiting ("The Adventures of Mercurius") and the numerous stories which so blantantly deal with sex, the pathology of love and the brittleness of the staunch bourgeois marital and familial rights ("The Gang of the Trunk"). The grotesques are not only verbal games which parody, under the guise of logic, the assiduous faith in ordered, logical reasoning; they also cajole the bourgeois by playing so lightheartedly with serious or taboo topics. Van Ostaijen summarizes his rebellion against seriousness, his defiance of bourgeois intolerance towards new and bold expressions in art which will not toe the moralistic line, in the following closing paragraph from a public address given in Brussels and Antwerp (1925–1926).[25] The career of Van Ostaijen and subsequent critical judgments only emphasize the myopic vision of the pedestrian mind, which could not see the courage of a man who had accepted the futility of life as a condition, and yet would not stoop to nihilism.

For all those available things: man's goodness, cleaner living and vegetarianism, the poverty of street-walkers as a springboard for the lyricism of poets who feel humane in a *tristitia post*-situation, the homeric battle with the lines wrought between eight and ten o'clock at night, humility or pride, the garret room or the Empire bed, all these things can not inspire me. Nor the cult of automobiles, airplanes or what one calls experiencing our roaring age. In short, all serious literature. Down with the sextons and with other ministers. Down with the improvement of mankind, but long live the improvement of racehorses! For, long live Pegasus, under the name of *Fox-trot* II.

THE STYLE OF THE GROTESQUES
A DESCRIPTION OF LINGUISTIC SUBVERSION

The prose style of Van Ostaijen generally encounters either critical praise or condemnation, with hardly any nuances between these two extremes. He is either lauded as a master of language with the poet's sensitivity for word and phrase, or he is dismissed as an unimpressive charlatan whose verbal inventiveness degenerates into tasteless puns. In both views the common denominator is that the style shows a highly cognizant employment of language. An examination of the stylistic and narrative characteristics will support the contention that this style is not a gratuitous acrostic diversion, but that the tales constitute, in fact, a subtle linguistic construction. They are examples of what Wolfgang Kayser called *das sprachliche Kunstwerk*. Kayser defines the verbal work of art as "[eine] in sich geschlossenes sprachliches Gefüge." The discussion may, perhaps, demonstrate how tightly knit these tales are and how the technical expertise proceeds to negate its own carefully constructed artifice.

ANARRATIVE NARRATIONS

Before examining the stylistic characteristics of Van Ostaijen's narrative prose, first a brief exposition of the tales' narrative structure. Generally speaking, the tales answer to at least the most basic requirements of the traditional story in having a protagonist and a rudimentary residue of dramatic action and narrative plot. There are a few which appear to be narrative trifles, lacking both a pronounced protagonist and a sharply delineated narrative pattern. Of these "anarratives" most examples date from the last four years of Van Ostaijen's career. *Clew of Ariadne (Kluwen van Ariadne)*, a collection of short pieces, was published in 1927. The unpublished pieces "Biological Delimitation of the Dancer" ("Biologische begrenzing van de danseur") and "This Isn't Funny at all" ("Dit is helemaal niet geestig") belong, from the point of view of style and content, to the same period as the afore mentioned collection. *Zoo for Children of*

Our Time (*Diergaarde voor kinderen van nu*), written in 1924, contains pieces ranging from two sentences to several pages in length, which may be seen as word-games, anecdotal fantasies or satirical notations devoid of such normative constants as plot and character. "The Ash" ("De Es") belongs to the same category. At a later stage it will become clear that these pieces share stylistic and conceptual characteristics with the major grotesques. They may be considered intermediary stages between the major tales and a small number of pieces, which evolved from peculiarities of style into what may be called abstract word paintings. Of the earlier works, one might consider including "The Marvelous Novel" ("De fijne roman"), "Between Fire and Water" ("Tussen Vuur en Water") and "Portrait of a Young Maecenas" ("Portret van een jonge meaceen") in this category, since they are, in terms of plot and character, tenuous narratives indeed. Still, these three pieces do deal with what might be conceived of as particular issues in a narrative fashion, though "Between Fire and Water," an evasive hybrid between essay and monologue, could not strictly be considered a narrative in the Aristotelian sense.

The bulk of these tales are designated as *grotesques*. Of these thirty tales one was conceived as a film scenario, "Bankruptcy Jazz" ("De Bankroet-Jazz"), and one, "The Gang of the Trunk" ("De Bende van de Stronk"), has the length of a novella. If the scenario is excluded as not properly belonging to the narrative genre, a body of twenty tales is left. From these twenty tales thirteen may be separated as major grotesques, because they seem to be either in a more finished or in a more accomplished form than the others. These thirteen tales are, in chronological order: "Claire's Herd or the Virginal Reveler" ("De kudde van Claire of de maagdelijke boemelaarster"), "The General" ("De Generaal"), "The Kept Hotel Key or the Small, Stupid Deed" ("De gehouden hotelsleutel of de kleine, domme daad"), "Mechtildis, That Good Girl" ("Mechtildis, die goede meid"), "The Prison in Heaven" ("Het gevang in de hemel"), "The Adventures of Mercurius, Corporation for the Exploitation of Counterfeiting" ("De lotgevallen van de Mercurius, maatschappij tot exploitatie der valse munterij"), "The City of Builders" ("De stad der opbouwers"), "The Fatal History of Scholem Weissbinder" ("De noodlottige geschiedenis van Scholem Weissbinder"), "Patriotism Incorporated" ("De Trust der Vaderlandsliefde"), "Ika Loch's Brothel" ("Het bordeel van Ika Loch"), "The Lost House Key" ("De verloren huissleutel"), and "The Gang of the Trunk" ("De Bende van de Stronk").

These thirteen tales either have a protagonist, or are primarily concerned with an invented narrative situation, or they include both these requirements of the short story. They have, ostensibly, a beginning, middle, and end. It is precisely with this generality that the Aristotelian norm ceases to function in the grotesques. An example are the beginnings. In most cases the first sentence introduces the protagonist in a somewhat laconic fashion.*

There was once a man who had spent twenty years in prison.
There was once a man who looked very distinguished.
One day I received from Scholem Weissbinder – in business and for casual acquaintances: Sam Weiss – a special delivery letter containing the following: "Come quickly. You are absolutely indispensable. Scholem."
Mister Hasdrubal Paaltjes was an Inspector of the Department of Bridges and Roads.
One could wonder why Claire at the age of eighteen was no longer under parental control.
For years Mechtildis had been selling her love in the Friedrichstrasse.

As these examples indicate, the introductory sentence invokes clearly and precisely what promises to be a perfectly succinct and straightforward narrative. This promise is never fulfilled. The author takes pleasure in luring the reader into this structural trap, where he remains caught in the mesh of paradox and subversive logic. The promise of normality dissolves in its antithesis: distortion. The beginning, in most cases, constitutes no more than one sentence or, at the most, one paragraph. Some beginnings, instead of introducing the protagonist, state a theme which will be amplified in the subsequent pages, where it will subordinate all other narrative props. Such beginnings are quite often a concept contrapuntal to the title, or develop a concept contained in the title in the body of the tale. Perhaps one might see these tales as prose applications of Van Ostaijen's poetic theory of *lyrisme à theme. Lyrisme à theme* is the formation of a poem by means of a series of associations developed from an initial phrase ("une phrase prémisse"). The "phrase prémisse . . . se développe d'une façon dynamique par les répercussions des mots dans le subconscient celui-ci livrera à la conscience la matière nécessaire à la continuation et à l'achèvement de l'édifice, tandis qu'en retour il sera du devoir de la conscience, de veiller à ce que cette matière reste dans les limites posées par la phrase prémisse."[1] An example of where this theory seems to have been applied to his prose work is the tale "The City of Builders." The "phrase prémisse" is included in the title, *opbouwen* "to build." The "reverberations" of this phrase call up a city, a city council with civic ardor, beautification of the city by building more and better. The "reverberations" also evoke the opposite of to build: to tear down. With these associations (one an antithesis) in mind, the story

* Translations in this chapter are as literal as possible in order to maintain the peculiar technical effects of Van Ostaijen's style.

("l'édifice") has obtained its material ("matière"). The city council votes a law into existence which threatens heavy punishment for anyone who dares tear down anything, and which rewards those who build. The city fathers are fanatical builders, and are soon carrying building to an extreme. What was once utilitarian becomes an absolute, "pure building," building "pour l'amour de l'art." (III, 142) Soon there is no more space to build, not even when one builds on top of older structures. The antithesis, which has been waiting in the wings, comes to the fore. An antibuilding movement is formed. The city fathers outlaw it and arrest its leader. They want a public execution to make an example of him, but there is no space for such an event. The leader of the anti-building movement is liberated, and the city fathers are deposed. The populace now clamors for open squares. A contiguous series (counterpointed by an antithesis which is a negative association) evolving from the original premise is developed into absurdity.

Throughout his theoretical writings on poetic theory, Van Ostaijen speaks of composition in terms which are analogous to Roman Jakobson's theory of metonymic art.[2] Van Ostaijen does not base his poetic theory (*lyrisme à theme*) on similarity, when the metaphor would be its most condensed expression, but on contiguity, on the aseity of the word, "par l'exactitude du choix de la place, par le choix de ses actions et de ses réactions, par l'assimilation de ses amitiés et le choc de ses inimitiés."[3] In other words, Van Ostaijen has chosen metonymic art, which is one of the two basic types of discourse which Roman Jakobson distinguishes in literary composition. Van Ostaijen's principle of association, basic to his *lyrisme à theme*, corresponds to Jakobson's principle of contiguity or *Berührungsassoziation*. The poem for Van Ostaijen is an independent organism, consisting of a chain of associatively connected realities. (IV, 130) Jakobson insists on the autonomy of the contiguously created *Verbindung*, which becomes an independent *Gegenstand*. These are not anarchic principles. For Van Ostaijen his *lyrisme à theme* is an "intellectual composition," subject to a "lyrical logic." (IV, 291) Metonymic art for Jakobson is the creative reflection of a modern philosophical preoccupation with *Gegenständlichkeit*. The grotesques of Van Ostaijen are sophisticated cerebral compositions, what Uyttersprot characterized as "verdichtete Logik." Though the principal preoccupation of the grotesques is logical reasoning, the net result, as in the case of "The City of Builders," is absurdity. The art of Van Ostaijen's grotesques is an art of contiguity; their method of reasoning is a contiguous ratiocination of an absurd logic. In Roman Jakobson's theory, metonymic art effaces the usual order of things so that an arbitrary contiguity becomes a causal sequence. Van Ostaijen's grotesques make use of a contiguous discourse to parody modern reliance on positivistic logic.

An instance of Jakobson's contiguity, or what Van Ostaijen calls "associatively connected realities" which "lie next to each other," (IV, 245) is a passage from the "The Lost House Key." The story's hero, Hasdrubal Paaltjes, has contracted syphilis. He consults a physician who, besides treatment, counsels continence or, as he calls it, following a "sexual diet."

Hasdrubal spoke the words after him. Sexual diet? Then a diet which was not sexual. Or how. What did they mean by this paradox? Distracted, lost in dreams. He felt like the captured eagle. Torturers and red-hot awls in the eyes. Inquisition. Was that a sexual diet. Hasdrubal understood: to keep to a diet or to commit suicide, this or that, but it was all the same. His fame: he never thought of a diet. He had to hold on to his fame. Taureau ardent. Torrent ardent. Sure. Women who had read stories of Indians called him that. To give up this fame was not all. This also meant making himself shamefully ridiculous. He had responsibilities to himself. That's the way it was: he was Hasdrubal.
   The diet appeared impossible.
   Come what may. Thus Paaltjes' fatalistic final sentence. And he behaved quite normally. Which for him, Paaltjes, was very normal. (III, 180)

The central point of the passage is Hasdrubal's sexual prowess and reputation. Continence is for him, as paradigmatic lover, a thought worse than death. The dilemma of continuing his sexual exploits, despite the contamination, or curing it by strict observance of his doctor's orders makes him feel, hyperbolically, like a chained eagle. Eagle associates with the chained Prometheus, and the torment of that mythological figure evokes the Inquisition. Through this contiguous chain, sexual continence is associated with the worst imaginable torture, if not suicide. His reputation is more important to Hasdrubal, and his self-glorification recalls the source of his fame: women. Associating his own epithets "ardent bull" and "ardent torrent" with women, he unwittingly provides a cynical comment on his lovers; these women revel in the juvenile literature of cowboys and indians. This satirical passage is a contiguous set of associations developed from the premise of Hasdrubal's hypertrophied sexuality. That it leads to Hasdrubal's conclusion not to suffer sexual dieting is not only skillfully established with a comic intention, but also represents the pivotal point of the story. Continuing his Don Juan existence despite his being the carrier of the syphilis spirochete marks the foundation of the luetic civilization of Megalopolis. This prose passage develops according to the principles of Van Ostaijen's *lyrisme à theme*. The premise is the counseled continence, which is developed contiguously (or by means of association as Van Ostaijen would have it) to Paaltjes' decision to behave as he would of old. The style of contiguity and the technique of metonymic art are the perfect implements for depicting the grotesque situation.

Another striking example illustrating the similarity between Van Ostaijen's *lyrisme à theme* and Jakobson's metonymic art is "The Sirens" ("De Sirenen"), which is discussed in more detail at a later stage. Suffice it to say here that the double meaning of the title (mythological figures and a modern acoustic instrument) is developed contiguously, without ever forcing a similarity which would destroy the ambivalence of the reciprocal replaceability of images in metonymic art. There are other instances where an opening premise is expanded contiguously. "Patriotism Incorporated" evolves from the opening phrase: "In illo tempore." "The Gang of the Trunk" also states its premise, the concept hypertrophy and its antithesis atrophy, in the first sentence. "Everyone knows those pedlars who are called Hidaljaneans after a one-sided hypertrophy, – which for the rest does not specify the nationality of these pedlars at all." (III, 51) The beginning of "Ika Loch's Brothel" takes a paragraph to set the tone of philosophical verbosity, of intellectualism, and of the inverse of logical inevitability, which is the subject of the tale. One may conclude that the beginning of these tales cannot be held responsible for their content and the course of their development.

The Aristotelian "middle" of a story is generally designated as the narrative proper. No matter how conventional some of the openings may be, the "middle" of a grotesque takes every possible liberty with the mechanics of narration. Distortion in terms of the narrative norm is most often represented by an atrophy of the story-line and a hypertrophy of exposition. An example is "The Gang of the Trunk," subtitled a "romantic story of robbery and love." This reminds one of a large territory of popular literature. The story proper starts in the third section, nine pages after the beginning. The hero Alessandro (the "stronk" = "trunk" of the title) is introduced on the second page, but only as a convenient starting point for a series of digressions and word-plays which do little to develop the character of the hero. Section II lectures on the superstition that deformed persons are supposed to have magical powers, especially in sexual matters. The entire third section, from a narrative point of view, establises nothing more than that in the capital of Atupal there is a rich nobleman (the ambassador from Hidaly) who resembles Alessandro to the point of also being a truncated man. In this manner Van Ostaijen, almost begrudgingly, keeps the bare outlines of the story going. This is obviously for ironic purposes; nothing resembles the rich staple of "drama" popular fiction thrives on. Here is an ironist playing with technique. There is for example in section eight, the wedding ceremony presided over by Cardinal Epernay. This should be a dramatic high point, since it represent the triumph of the deception; the pseudo-Marquis de Mirlitonare marries the most eligible debutante of the capital, thereby sealing the success of the gang's criminal mission. However, the ceremony and its principals are hardly mentioned, and the section turns out to be a long diatribe on marriage. The honeymoon, in stories of this type a particularly rewarding experience, is dealt with as follows: "Honeymoon, taking off." (III, 92) The description of the mariage becomes a satiric testimonial, anti-Freud; psychology and psychoanalysis are reasoned into absurdity. The stereotype of the romantic popular novel has been negated.

Another example of this subversion of plot and narrative convention is "Claire's Herd." The opening sentence asks the question why Claire at eighteen, is no longer subject to parental authority. More than three pages later, the author reiterates the same statement with the "clarification" that his readers no longer need to take it as impossible that Claire, at eighteen, was no longer subject to parental control. At the same time he negates the divergences between the first and second statements with the *non sequitur*: "Since I have never questioned this fact, it was easy for me to invent this introduction." (III, 292) The long digression was built on a series of elaborations and rhetorical discourses about words and ideas implied by previous sentences. Women, men (and the species of the genus: Claire's mother and father), age, domestic life and other subjects related to marriage are discussed with a humor couched in reflective exposition. Parenthetically, it might be noted that this is yet another instance of Van Ostaijen's use of contiguity as it was discussed in the case of "The City of Builders" and "The Lost House Key." Meanwhile, one suddenly realizes that nothing essential has been said about fictional parents; essential, that is, for normal dramatic and narrative purposes. Instead, one is introduced to Claire's private world, a nightclub milieu of such anti-social characters as *vieux-marcheurs* (or gay, old blades) and *rastas* (an abbreviation of *rastaquouères* or parvenus). The expected does not materialize. The opportunity to exploit a situation ready-made for popular novels, of a young innocent girl amidst unsavory characters in a dangerous environment, becomes a lengthy discours on what constitutes the difference between a *rasta* and a *vieux-marcheur*.

The story of the exiled Peruvian General in "The General" is a thirty-page discourse on the philosophy of war and eroticism. A potentially lurid potboiler like "The Lost House Key," dealing with venereal disease, is an objective account written in a formal style, of how this social stigma becomes the cultural pride of a metropolis. Perhaps "Ika Loch's Brothel" carries the narrative anti-norm to its extreme. Whatever preconceptions or expectations one might have on that topic, they never materialize. The tale is perhaps the most sterilized brothel story one might ever encounter. In fact, it is a lengthy series of philosophical discussions and expositions on sundry matters, which, in a gratuitous manner, happen to be related to the business of running a brothel. There are other tales, such as "The Prison in Heaven" and "The Kept Hotel Key," where one might speak of a more direct narrative development. But even in these examples digressions and word-games are abundant. They usually begin with an antithetical situation, which is developed *ad absurdum*. The released prisoner pines away for prison life in "The Prison in Heaven." A man, tormented by suicidal tendencies, kills himself in order to escape committing suicide in "The Fatal History of Scholem Weissbinder." Afraid of the dangers of speed, a man kills himself to avoid being killed in an express train in "The Conviction of Notary Telleke." In "The Kept Hotel Key" the main character systematically banishes love from his world only to be foiled by the affectionate misunderstanding of his wife, and commits suicide to escape the dilemma of his guilt.

In most of these tales, the traditional narrative norm is undermined. Many grotesques are subversions of the bourgeois novel. Whatever common, popular taste might expect of an imaginative work of prose is skillfully withheld. Little resemblance to real life is left. Van Ostaijen makes a point of being indifferent to quotidian reality, to commonplaces, to the accepted norm of popular taste. Narrative coherence is dissolved. "Intermezzo" discusses this dichotomy between the grotesque's metonymic technique and popular taste. The mutinous audience in the cosmic playhouse asks exactly for what the grotesque can never given them. "Away with the grotesque. Real true life. Like so and so, or like thus and so. They are playwrights. Hooray! a grotesque is only grotesque because it itself is grotesque. A grotesque lacks coherence. And coherence c'est le nerf de l'art." (III, 199) Such an accusation has often been levelled at Van Ostaijen. A sober realist fails to see a definite congruity in these tales: a metonymic coherence. The world and the style of the grotesques create their own laws according to grotesque standards. Roman Jakobson emphasizes how an arbitrary contiguity is accepted as an autonomous causality. "Die geschaffene Verbindung wird an und für sich zum Gegenstand."

The heroes of these tales are also contrary to popular preconceptions. Characterization is atrophied. They are not E. M. Foster's "well-rounded characters" but linear, narrative etchings drawn with verbal nuances. In

"Intermezzo" the director answers the charge that his heroes are not in accordance with the popular ideal with the telling reply that such an observation is quite correct.

I also know that the heroes I have shown up till now, are not absolute concretizations of the heroic ideal. But why do my heroes have to be heroes? Is a fusion of hero and harlequin not much more interesting? You probably also think that my heroes have been all too wretchedly copied from the same pattern. If this is your opinion then I am forced to attribute it to an uncultivated sensuality. Then you don't understand nuances, nor the differences which an etching-needle mind does understand. Or might my heroes be unnatural? In my panopticon nothing is unnatural, ladies and gentlemen, if only by hypothesis. At the most, contrary to nature. (III, 200)

As Wolfgang Kayser points out in his book on *Das Groteske in Malerei und Dichtung*, the artists of the grotesque prefer the linear media of the visual arts. As examples one could point to the etchings of Callot, Goya and Ensor. The curious paradox inherent in the graphic medium is that, despite its relative size and lacking the impact of colors, as in oils, it nevertheless invokes a proximity which can be at times uncomfortably familiar. This "Distanzlosigkeit" of graphics ensures a "ganz-darin-Sein." [4] Yet the paradox remains that the graphic medium cannot achieve as full-bodied a representation as a painting can; that is to say, from the point of view of realism. The graphic figures, with their own uncanny life, are on intimate footing with us, but are deficient in "realism." Speaking of Breughel's graphic art, Van Ostaijen distinguishes between Breughel's simplicity and Rembrandt's pathos. Breughel, according to Van Ostaijen, sees the blank paper as fundamental synthesis which need hardly be touched by the pen to call forth the "pre-existing object" embedded in it. Contour and shape are not objects in themselves, but merely accentuation and decoration of this fundamental synthesis. One could draw an analogy to the grotesques. The world is the paper on which the artist need hardly trace his pen to portray its essential grotesque quality. Van Ostaijen can therefore insist that his heroes are not unnatural, since nature is the "pre-existent object," and his fictional portraits mere visualizations of a fundamental reality. His heroes do not need bold strokes from the fictional brush to call them to life. The *a priori* grotesqueness of the world is so potent that the nuances drawn by the mind's etching-needle suffice to convey his essential vision of a world out of joint. Hence the unity of style and theme of his grotesques is produced by Van Ostaijen's innate experience of the world as absurdity. The stylistic components, the characters, the images are all metonymic formulations of this basic unity.

A graphic example of this principle is Promethea, the mysterious Venus of "Ika Loch's Brothel," who definitely seems to have been drawn with a narrative etching-needle. She is, in fact, a sum of nuances. Promethea is the physical superlative of the establishment, the prime attraction for the customers. But the description of her is a feat of understatement, of suggestion. No bold strokes to present a lascivious portrait befitting a wanton setting and a lewd narrative. Promethea, in this strangest of all lubricious tales, acquires verisimilitude through addition, a sum of graphic distinctions, of fine nuances which presents a negation of eroticism. Promethea is a "harmony of barely shown things." (III, 119) But the descriptive nuances do not imply nuances of characterization. We know nothing of Promethea as a person; she remains a mystery. Promethea is an absolute of beauty, but she bears no resemblance to the popular notion of a prostitute; ultimately she is anti-erotic. A tentative assertion might conclude that most of the characters are either a-human and bear little resemblance to traditional protagonists, or they are helpless tools in a metaphysical game in which the odds are overwhelmingly against them.

Action, another major narrative element, is also curtailed in these tales. In grotesques like "Ika Loch's Brothel," "The General," "Claire's Herd," "Mechtildis, That Good Girl," dramatic action has been virtually eliminated. In others, action is constantly syncopated by the discursive digressions, rendering it very brittle indeed. From a normative view of fiction, the lenght of these tales is unnecessary for the development of the plot. Not does the dramatic action lead, in most cases, to an expected climax. Either the tale is ended with a narrative *non sequitur,* or the hero has vanished in the course of the tale, and one is left with a narrative vacuum where the hero should have been. The ending more often than not only opens into innumerable questions, and concludes very little. Many times endings are enigmatic and abrupt, and contradict the elaborate verbal construction which they foreclose. At the end of "The Gang of the Trunk" one becomes involved in dialectical arguments concerning a legacy and the fraud which has been perpetrated, but no more is heard from the principals; they seem to have vanished behind a smokescreen of words. In "Ika Loch's Brothel," a tale which lives a precarious narrative existence from the beginning, Ika Loch disappears, and the brothel is reduced to a punctilious description of the furnishings and the poetic mystery of "a nightvase with a deep red rose." In "The Lost House Key," the hero Hasdrubal Paaltjes, has been superseded long before the end by lengthy intellectual theories concerning the reasons why or how Paaltjes lost his house key. Another type of ending, equally abrupt, is sober and concrete, and therefore, antithetical to the absurd development of the tale.

A preliminary investigation into the general aspects of this narrative fiction has established a number of observations. Negatively, these tales are a criticism and a denial of popular taste and popular fiction. They destroy the continuity and the presuppositions of the bourgeois novel through a hypertrophy of structural freedom and an atrophy of the narrative norm. These tales are technically defiantly autonomous and critical of conventions. The author has taken a position of consequent objectivity, concomitant with a fictional world where all things narrative are equal. One could call it a position of creative indifference. The aberrations of the narrative norm are not random distortions, but result from a theoretical presupposition of absolute liberty of the narrative structure. Plot, unity of action, characterization are subverted and distorted. When these conventional props have been removed, what remains as the content of these tales? Their content is syntax; language equals content. For a writer such as Van Ostaijen who practices metonymic art in both poetry and prose, the fictional world is created in such a way that for him, in Roman Jakobson's words ". . . jedes Zeichen, jedes geschaffene Wort mit einer vollen selbständigen Realität ausgestattet ist und die Frage nach seinem Bezug zu irgend einem aussenliegenden Gegenstand, ja die Frage der Existenz eines solchen Gegenstandes wird volkommen überflüssig." The content and subject matter of Van Ostaijen's grotesques are subordinate to style and form. Language and thought are the building materials for these verbal constructions. But language and thought are used antithetically to their normal intentions; language painstakingly formulates the irrational, while thought relentlessly pursues its opposite, cancellation of the rational.

One final general feature of these tales remains to be discussed. If nothing else, all the grotesques are highly cerebral narratives. This predominant intellectuality is characteristic of Van Ostaijen and of his times. Quite early in his career Van Ostaijen's comments on contemporary art stressed the cerebral character of his own generation of artists. Almost at the same time he was forced to defend this position. The article in which he did so, dating from 1917 when he had just turned twenty-one, used Gleizes and Metzinger's *Du 'Cubisme'* for his defence. The pivotal idea of Cubism, according to the two painter-apologists, was that ". . . le monde visible ne devient le monde réel que par l'opération de la pensée, et que les objets qui nous frappent avec le plus de force ne sont pas toujours ceux dont l'existence est la plus riche en verités plastiques." [5] This stern emphasis on the cerebral basis and possibilities of art was developed by Van Ostaijen in his first major essay of 1918, "Expressionism in Flanders" ("Expressionisme in Vlaanderen"). According to Van Ostaijen, one of the most cogent features of the simultaneous explosion of Cubism in France, Expressionism in Germany, and Futurism in Italy is its anti-materialistic, cerebral and spiritual program. In short, the new art is a turning away from the traditional "physioplasticity" to "ideoplasticity." (IV, 19) "Ideoplasticity" is a theoretical *leitmotiv* throughout his speculative writings, is a concise summation of his poetic intentions, and is most certainly an accurate description of the grotesques. As fictional formulations of a modern "ideoplastic" movement, the grotesques are indispensable units for the understanding of Van Ostaijen's total literary design. Again, in a discussion of the sculpture by the Flemish artist Oskar Jespers, he concludes that this is a form of art which elicits the impression of being purely mental. Cubism, he states in his essay "What Is Wrong with Picasso" ("Wat is er met Picasso"), "moved from the emotionally rational to the consciously-rational." (IV, 80) Poetry is "a lyrically intuitive conversion of epistemology; that along with the experience of the phenomenon tree I can also experience my conception of this tree as a phenomenon." (IV, 119)

The accent on cerebrality, on the controlling intellect, is more prominent in the essays on art than in those on poetry. But this is only because the formulations concerning poetry try to explain what a poem should be, what constitutes a poem. Dealing with creative inspiration and with the meaning of lyricism, Van Ostaijen grappled with problems and areas of the human spirit which may be almost immune to ratiocination. The fact remains that, notwithstanding the Pythian nature of poetry, Van Ostaijen constantly ventured to wed inspiration to intellect, to wed Apollo to Athena. Prosodic innovations by Van Ostaijen were built on a foundation of intellectual and conscious control; built on a logic of poetic construction. The very term "organic prosody," for example, contains a demand for structure, for meaningful relationships between units of tone, of linguistic tension and linguistic chromatics. A poem for Van Ostaijen develops logically from a premise, while the associative reverberations that this premise evokes are constructed contiguously into a pattern in a lyrico-logical manner, which motivates the formulation of the subconscious premise into a poetic structure. The occasional rebukes of experimentation which his work must still endure are somewhat puzzling to an attentive reader of Van Ostaijen. On the contrary, there was something of the pedagogue, if not a touch of the pedant, in Van Ostaijen the theorist. An artist first, to be sure, he labored most of his later years to write a sort of handbook which would explain his audacious lyrical alchemy to a dull-witted audience. "Cubism is no longer only an artistic and plastic concern. It is first and foremost an architectonic concern: to create a new style. A new esthetic scholasticism, if you like. A bas l'anarchie. Away with the good taste of the subject as norm. Laws. Precise, tangible things. In short, away with the artist." (IV, 11)

An esthetic scholasticism. Not only was the intellect a basis for Van Ostaijen's own endeavors, but also the dominant force in contemporary movements in art. Reason, intellect, logic, mathematical construction, the *ens rationis* reverberates throughout the 1920's. Theo van Doesburg, the leader of "De Stijl" movement reiterates this opinion in his articles for the periodical *De Stijl*. "For the same reason that the poets shall arrive at a new poetry, the thinkers shall become conscious of their original task: the search for the reasonableness and functionality of life, in order to determine therefrom the systematization of life's construction." [6] Vassily Kandinsky insists that modern art strives "zum Nicht naturellen, Abstrakten und zu innerer Natur." [7] Piet Mondriaan went beyond the cubistic credo and its relatively representational objects to acknowledge only a strict, stern, spiritual discipline and a mathematically precise method of art to ward off any impending charms nature might lure him with. Apollinaire in his manifesto "L'Esprit Nouveau et les Poètes," published in 1918, stresses the spirit of discipline as well as the marvels of the new age. "C'est pourquoi l'esprit nouveau se réclame avant tout de l'ordre et du devoir qui sont les grandes qualités classiques par quoi se manifeste le plus hautement l'esprit français, et il leur adjoint la liberté."

Van Ostaijen was a child of his time, and it was the mind which was adventurous in the arts and did not allow the emotions to gain the upper hand. The senses were not denigrated, as Van Ostaijen's poetry clearly shows. But the new age, with its chain-reaction of revolutionary discoveries and events, challenged creative spirits to formulate a new notation for the music of modern times. Instead of an emotional anarchy, man's intellect accepted the challenge; the "new spirit" was a spirit of creative intellectuality. The cerebrality of the grotesques, therefore, is not only natural to Van Ostaijen's personality and style, but also indicative of the formal spirit of the contemporary artistic revolution. That Van Ostaijen makes use of cerebrality to castigate a fraudulent ratiocination of a world turned topsy-turvy does not hide the fact that intellect parries intellectuality in a contest of keen wit. The grotesques are neither popular fiction nor a game of literary blindman's buff, but products of erudition: they are games of logic. Michelangelo wrote a terse motto for the modern movement: "Si pinge col cervello, non con la mano." It is also an apt aphorism for the style of Van Ostaijen's grotesques.

SYNTAX AS MEANING

A discussion of the syntactical elements of these tales will belie Stuiveling's accusation (among others) that these tales are little more than gratuitous experimentations. After a process of elimination one question remains. What constitutes the content of these tales when most conventional props of the narrative structure have atrophied? The answer seems to come from the implication that, when the narrative features have been stripped, only one component of fiction is left: language. In accordance with this assumption, the syntactical elements will be examined on the basis of fairly traditional usage, in order to indicate literary antecedents and to disprove critical contentions of arbitrary experimentation. A guideline may be provided by Van Ostaijen's own pronouncements on prose style. Unfortunately, he rarely expressed himself on this topic with the same vehemence or fullness as on poetic theory. However, in a little known review he outlines very briefly the following factors for prose style. He legislates that syntax equals content. Sentences should be constructed from contrapuntal formations, and their rhythm syncopated to provide contrast within the sentence unit and to undermine continuity. He upholds repetition as a major rhetorical device, and he recommends sparseness for sentences, concluding paragraphs, as well as entire stories.[8] Three major uses of language can be isolated from this brief pronouncement by Van Ostaijen: syntactical deformation, repetition and contradiction. These three general devices are also basic to metonymic art. In his essay on Pasternak, Jakobson speaks of stylistic *Zersetzung,* even at the price of catachresis, the reciprocity of images, and of contradiction inherent in his types of *Berührungsassoziationen.* These three fundamentals will be discussed in terms of a series of specific rhetorical applications in Van Ostaijen's prose style. Argumentation will be discussed as a major technique in these grotesques, and the section closes with a note on diction.

But first a general view of the style, with two random samples. Van Ostaijen's sentences are generally loose and lengthy, and may be classified as non-periodic sentences. Verbose, and anything but succinct, their rhythm is broken (syncopated) to obtain an even more languid effect. The verb seems subordinate to a succession of nouns and adjectives. The sentences are highly predicative and their subject often elusive. This creates an intentionally abstruse effect.

After the novelist in some hundreds of pages has told everything about his heroes, that he has five buttons on his vest and she breasts which are not voluptuous besides a nervousness which manifests itself in her always wanting to stick her

10 fingers in the marmeladejar, after having told all this circumstantially, the novelist ends with the axiom that one cannot tell the ending.

In this example the long parenthetical phrase slows down the rhythm of the sentence, a deceleration which grinds to a halt with the syllogistic end, mocking and denigrating the entire sentence, not only in terms of content, but also through its syntactical position.

I thought it would appear quite normal, if I explained the estrangement between husband and wife in this manner; furthermore the forty-five year old merchant who, after a marriage of eighteen years, felt he should not onesidedly pass by the other possibilities of life, appeared to me to be a decent burgher of novel society.

This sentence could easily, without harming grammar or content, be divided into two separate ones. Linking them together with a semicolon gives the intended ponderous, rhetorical effect of a treatise or a learned dissertation. The second half of the sentence shows a hyperbatic effect; the last phrase should come after "merchant." The effect of the hysteron proteron is one of ironic emphasis here; the bourgeois image of the husband is subtly undermined with a charge of infidelity, slipped in almost unnoticed before the final concepts of popular normality: "decent," "burgher," "novel society."

Both sentences refuse to admit a precise syntactical conclusion. They exemplify a process of analysis which does not resolve, but leaves its subject dissected, vulnerable and footloose. It is an analytical rhetoric, which fails to draw definite conclusions. And if it seems to follow a logical course (usually in cases where the initial premise was antithetical to normality to begin with), it analyzes itself logically into absurdity. Each sentence is an argumentation. Indeed, each tale is an argumentation which could be succinct, but seldom is. Scholarly and academic argumentation tends to prefer slow, parenthetical constructions. An argument often uses rhetorical figures. Van Ostaijen's style in these tales is an elaborate rhetoric that proceeds preferably by disorder, by defect, by the hyperbatic process. Such a practice indicates a negative intent, indicates deformation, indicates the ubiquity in this style of the principles of atrophy and hypertrophy and ultimately indicates cerebrality. Instead of compiling statistical examples from all the stories, it is more palatable to examine one tale, and pursue a number of specific rhetorical devices which are departures from the grammatical or syntactical norm. "Ika Loch's Brothel" is a good example since, in many ways, it epitomizes the form of narrative under discussion.

Deformation

The style of the grotesques which often seems quite odd, makes use of such traditional rhetorical figures as anastrophe, hypallage, hyperbaton, zeugma, polyptoton, and many others. The rhetorical figures used here are traditional and formal in their usage. To base a discussion of a modern author's style on historical usage might seem fortuitous. However, it was done deliberately to describe a style with many formal rhetorical elements which, in their new context, become a modern rhetoric. This system of rhetorical figures was, after all, a rigorous and highly cerebral one. As a basis for comparison, in order to establish the skill and sophistication of Van Ostaijen's style, one can hardly find a more appropriate system. The discussion of individual elements is based on an examination of the traditional rhetoric in Shakespeare's work by Sister Miriam Joseph, *Shakespeare's Use of the Arts of Language* (New York, 1949). One of the basic characteristics of this style is syntactical deformation, dislocation of normal wordorder. The following sentences are some extreme examples.

After an effort that was short and easy like every routine that develops in a natural and progressive manner by itself, the madam Ika Loch was at the head of a firstclass brothel, a business which soon operated on a respectable credit-balance.
Not fear, but rather a purely intellectual respect had Ika Loch for these laws which she, in her function as directress, had to submit to.
Polka was Ika Loch the most beautiful dance.
Too bad, that without more ado the objects to which the diagram had to be supplied, were not very pleased with it.
An end was she.

A frequent syntactical aberration in this prose is a deformation whereby, as Sister Miriam Joseph puts it, "the application of words is perverted and sometimes made absurd." Van Ostaijen obtains unusual effects by forcing abnormal relationships between words in the syntactical unit.

Sharply and exactly weighed the necklace throat against body.
Her slightly curved lines faded into the thin capacity of her sicklelegs; the burden of the small body was almost too heavy for them.
And it happened often that she was not wrong.

Parenthetical constructions, in which the sentence is broken by interposing clauses, phrases or words, are common.

. . . immediately Ika Loch is present and inspects the client, which is strange behavior for a madam, especially since . . .
But she did not allow herself to be disturbed by this and sincerely pitied these

stupid clients, who still, against their own advantage, stubbornly claimed to know better.

This had to be, she felt, correct.

A recurring dislocation of the syntactical norm is the omission of words which are not readily supplied by the reader. Reminiscent of ellipsis, the omission is usually abrupt which adds a strongly syncopated rhythm to the sentence.

From the point of view of fertility already sexless.
That Promethea very beautiful, Ika Loch recognized, but as to the content . . .
Besides whether he was a jockey or not no one has ever been able to establish; a sex murderer, yes – but this not as a social status.
. . . this masterpiece had Ika Loch managed to accomplish to eliminate the essential desire, to suppress the sex drive in sexual life.

The following two sentences are examples of the traditional figure of ellipsis.

The rooms on the first floor were properly bourgeois; those on the second floor more elementary furnished, though no less spic and span.
The washstand in a room on the first floor was porcelain, on the second it was enamel, usually white with not too garish little flowers.

Van Ostaijen's style often includes Germanisms. The following example includes a typically German practice of delaying the verb till the end of the sentence. It also employs a minor rhetorical device called polysyndeton, which uses many conjunctions to produce a slow, deliberate effect.

. . . that it, literally, requires a *super*human power Ika Loch psychologically pure, only and directly from her own specificity, without the indirect path via the reactions of the outside world, that is to say esoterically to present.

Repetition

Two main features of both argumentation and style remain to be discussed. Repetition and contrast are perhaps the two archetypal structures of language, basic to stylistic inventiveness and the development of an argument. The obvious figures of repetition, anaphora and epistrophe, are hardly ever employed by Van Ostaijen. Usually the subtler uses, reminiscent of syllogistic reasoning, or a cerebral playing with words are evident in Van Ostaijen's style. His poetic practice gave him a keen sense of the ambiguity of words and their ability to assume a life of their own.

A form of repetition which turns a sentence or clause around, a grammatical inversion akin to logical conversion, is antimetabole. An example of what might be considered an extension of antimetabole can be found in the tale "The General." The General feels that the saying "Si vis pacem, para bellum" is a slogan for artificial militarism and has, therefore, no relationship to true martiality. Militarism dampens the martial spirit of a nation, domesticates it as it were. The General reasons that if the draft were abolished and peace were profound and lasting, the basic drive for war (= pure martiality) would rise even stronger in nations. On the basis of this argument he feels that the slogan should be: "Si vis bellum, para pacem." In the same tale, the General bemoans the fate of pure warfare. At the present time, he argues, war is an economic tool, and its philosophy is summed up in the maxim: "L'argent c'est le nerf de la guerre." But since he posits war for war's sake, the General rewrites the maxim as "La guerre c'est le nerf de l'argent."

Another kind of repetition used by Van Ostaijen is the rhetorical device of polyptoton. Polyptoton is, strictly speaking, a rhetorical figure which repeats a word in different cases or inflexions in the same sentence. In this style one may perhaps speak of an extended application, where polyptoton may also include a repetition of components shared by a series of words, a repetition with change.

She had made unlucky change into a chanceless norm.
... and this new life they proudly called the sexual cerebral sex life ...
Besides, whether he was a jockey no one has ever been able to establisch; a sex murderer, yes – but this not as a social standing. This murder, though, was more than sufficient to shock Ika Loch. One did certainly not come to a brothel to commit murder, but, as she put it, to amuse oneself. And what the police were saying about a sex murder remained incomprehensible to her.
... reaction rather than action was given ...
... one could assume that she was only an illusion – as a madam, sexual delusion.

Van Ostaijen was also fond of using a series of words which are closely related in meaning, but not quite synonyms. A series of words which are juxtaposed in this manner in terms of meaning, gives the sentence the accumulated effect of repetition. The syntax of such sentences seems to be subordinated to this series of repetitive juxtapositions.

Promethea! barely and briefly her fingers touched the veil, lightly pushing it aside, that was already sufficient ...
Her slightly curved lines faded into the thin capacity of her sicklelegs; the burden of the small body was almost too heavy for them. The air around them too heavily charged, it seemed as if the legs, in a last effort, were for a moment still perfectly beautiful, before they sprung under the pressure of these opposing energies.
The fact however that most of the whores were crippled as she was, made her strongly believe that the others were defective.

Iteration is a characteristic feature of this style. The same word will be repeated again and again if it is germane to the development of an argumentative paragraph, the subject of a passage, or to an entire tale. In "Ika Loch's Brothel," the word "authoritarian" recurs throughout the tale, as if to emphasize the legality and authority of Ika Loch's obverse logic, to the point of being used five times in one paragraph. In one sentence the word "scepticism" is repeated three times. When Ika Loch's authority is firmly established on matters sexual, the word "subconscious" occurs several times in succession. It reoccurs, along with its contextual synonym "sex life," in a passage disclosing that Ika Loch has been sterile since her teens; there are obvious ironic overtones. Hence iteration serves a definite stylistic purpose: to underline intended irony in a subtle, unobtrusive fashion, or aids in pursuing a line of argumentation by reiterating a particular (usually abstract) word or concept.

Contradiction

Contradiction is another major device in this cerebral, skillfully constructed "sprachliches Kunstwerk." Contradiction provides tension. In Van Ostaijen's prose style contradiction is usually of a subtle nature, which might escape a casual reader, but which tends to build towards a cumulative effect of estrangement and invalidation of the tale's logical argument. An example of an elaborate series of contradictions can be seen in Ika Loch's scheme for matching the clients with her girls. The scheme is devoid of nuances; a contradiction in terms since a scheme should properly account for a series of degrees between two extremes. Her matchmaking is not based on the principle of like to like, but on that of contradiction. A privative term is maintained here, in that by definition matchmaking seeks to exclude contradictory principles by matching correlatives. The sentence which follows this schematic prognostication is, formally speaking, litotes (a thought expressed by denying its contrary), which subverts Ika Loch's argumentation: "And it happened often that she was not mistaken."

The effect of Ika Loch's system is further negated when one reads after a series of scientific terms (*authoritarian, system, principle, data*), that her success barely edged the level of purely accidental luck. Here the contradiction is couched in terms of a paradox; her system is only relatively successful by virtue of chance. Then follows the exhibition of the principle of contradiction in her system of matchmaking: corpulent men, she legislates, like svelte women; barely fullgrown girls are for epicurean old men; teenage boys appreciate hefty females. This systematic application of a popular belief is negated (contradicted) by the subjects of the system, who show tastes contradictory to the belief which Ika Loch has elevated to an axiom. This exclusion of nuances in her system precipitates near financial disaster for her establishment. A fat man is matched with a skinny woman and rebels against the choice; as a bone merchant he has seen too many skeletons. A high school teacher is not a refined connoisseur, but is basic and instinctual in his appetites. Undismayed, Ika Loch quickly assumes this inverted state of affairs as axiomatic. And so the series of contradictions (paradoxes, privative comparisons, relatives, and so on) are continued *ad absurdum*. What started as a system of contradictions based on a popular belief becomes an axiomatic application of incongruity, which in turn could also be inverted to suit a different purpose. Style and content are like a madly spinning top which the author could keep going for as long as he wishes.

Paradox and incongruity are the creative principles of these tales, and one can never predict when or how a series of contradictions will be stopped. This can be seen in the tale under discussion. The contradictory nature of Ika Loch's scheme reverberates through the tale until it echoes absurdity. The very inability to define correctly the clients' wishes is seen by them as indicative of her superior knowledge concerning her profession. A sex murder reinforces the clients' opinion that Ika Loch's authoritarian behavior masks a superior, scientific knowledge of their sexual appetites. This absurd train of thought is pursued with rigorous logic by those customers who declare fidelity to her principles. Ika Loch's establishment becomes a landmark in the city, where it is the only brothel which serves its customers on a "scientific" basis. At this point the author discloses that Ika Loch is totally asexual, physically as well as psychologically. If anything, she is cerebral. But even her cerebrality is of a highly dubious nature since she elevates chance occurrence to axiomatic truth. Yet the story tells us that Ika Loch is an expert on sexual matters, that she is a widely acclaimed authority on applying psychoanalytic methods to sexual desires, and that her establishment is of unique service to the town. At the same time, a set of contradictions runs counter to these discoveries. This paradigm of sexual expertise is basically cerebral, as opposed to emotional and instinctual drives. She is myopic, which makes it very difficult for her to see clearly the people she is supposed to match, while her success is rooted in plain and simple luck. Such a progression of contradictions is not only acceptable, but successful within the autonomous world of the grotesque. This is "supreme logical disorder, the acceptance of a contradiction," as Sister Miriam Joseph puts it, advanced with resolute reasoning. Contradiction is the conceptual and stylistic manifestation of the bifold authority of atrophy and hypertrophy.

As was previously indicated, the principle of contradiction is not only applied generically, but also specifically. Within one sentence, unexpected contrasts may quite often occur: "From this there now followed the present state of affairs that she, the madam of a brothel, did not have the slightest notion of sex, indeed she simply could not understand the urge." There is a perfect formal antithesis in the sentence: "Promethea's immobility in death was equal to her contained peace in life." The skill of the stylistic architecture of these tales becomes clearer when one notices how this particular sentence refers back to the curious description of Promethea on the preceding page. The accent in that description was on the a-human aspect of Promethea's beauty. This was beauty as an end in itself. Promethea was a principle, not a living entity: "An end was she." Promethea was a paradigmatic occurrence, devoid of life and humanity, a conceptual absolute of beauty constructed out of verbal nuances. She too, like Ika Loch, was sexless. This perfection of idealized beauty is absurdly incongruous as the attraction of a brothel. If Ika Loch is hypertrophied intellect, then Promethea is hypertrophied beauty; both are equally deficient in normality and humanity. Both are extremes in the story's anti-world. This contradiction of paradigmatic beauty in such a "realistic" institution as a brothel provokes a tension, a fearful estrangement. The effect of *Verfremdung* is only underlined by her death. The lifelessness of Promethea, which was implied in the description of her, is echoed and realized in the description of the rigidity of her dead body. In death she is still as inanimate and ideal a composition as she was in life. Her corpse is described with the same subtle nuances of color as when she first appeared as the brothel's prime attraction. This is an example of how contradiction and repetition are basic to the construction of a conceptual incongruity in an inverted world.

Two other aspects of contradiction and repetition are fundamental to the stylistic formation of these tales. One is the use of antonyms within the same sentence or set of sentences.

From the point of view of fertility, already sexless.
To wear dull black and brilliant orange was, according to her, Promethea's most outstanding feature.
. . . the inversely determined success . . .
. . . Promethea had torn the grey web from his intoxication and contrasted sharply glittering orange silk and, tormentingly, her navel was still with illusionary peace.

A modification of contradiction is the practice of concluding a long paragraph with a brief sentence; a practice reminiscent of the larger narrative structure, where an entire tale is concluded with a short, laconic sentence. Usually the brevity of the sentence contracts a lengthy argument into a pithy, equivocal statement, which pushes the illogical logic of the preceding argumentation to its nth degree of absurdity. "Polka was Ika Loch the most beautiful dance," concludes a discourse of a scientific nature (including mathematical equations) on the premise that cleanshaven gentlemen, if not perverse, are at least subtle in their sexuality. The next paragraph, which analyzes the dissolution of Ika Loch's system of matchmaking, ends with the succinct reminder of disaster: "Furious, everybody left the brothel." The description of Promethea, which presents her as an abstraction and as an ideal, concludes: "An end was she." A series of paragraphs, which describe not only Ika Loch's success as a madam, but also her totally erroneous conclusions about her customers' desire, ends with: "The scientific and objective judgment of Ika Loch." The entire story concludes with the brief and enigmatic sentence: "This room was reserved for important guests."

ARGUMENTS OF ABSURDITY

The tales in general and paragraphs in particular may be seen as argumentations or as logical demonstrations. Most characters, when they hold forth, indulge in lengthy discourses to prove the normality of their incongruous positions and convictions. Demonstration is executed in a process of logical progression, and one must remember that the reasoning perpetrated in these tales is perfectly congruous within the autonomy of the story. It becomes incongruous when readers, being outsiders to this world, oppose it to the reality in which they live. Yet the reasoning seems plausible, because it is based on certain modes of thought and concepts familiar to us. If this were not so, we would be in the domain of fairy tales. The grotesques do not belong to this type of fiction, because they share a basis of familiarity with the reader's world and experience. As a dispassionate observer, knowing the distinction between reality and absurdity, the reader may judge the arguments to be syllogistic; a fallacious reasoning which results in incongruity. But one must always remember that Ika Loch would be shocked if her train of thought were condemned as such. Yet the fact remains that the world of Ika Loch, the world of logic, constantly sins against logic.

In logicam peccare, to sin against logic, could be the motto of these tales. Naturally, examples can be found in all of them. Again, this discussion restricts itself to "Ika Loch's Brothel." Everything happens contrariwise in this tale. The customers of Ika Loch's establishment will not comply with her axiomatic reasoning that one can direct a brothel on the assumption that opposites are attractive to each other. A man is fat. All fat men like thin women. Ergo, this fat customer wants this thin prostitute. Reality refutes the syllogism. The fat customer is a bone merchant, and he is sick of looking at skeletons. Logic and existence confront each other as polar principles and refuse to be analogous. Similar occurrences combine to provoke a rebellion by the customers against Ika Loch's axiomatic thinking. But then the tide of opinion turns again in a most curious fashion. One day a murder is committed in the brothel. The crime is strange and is never explained. This, one would assume, would inhibit frequentation of a potentially dangerous place. But the crime turns out to be a welcome advertisement which fate (luck) extended *gratis* to Ika Loch. The crime, paradoxically enough, brings the rebels back to the fold. Now Ika Loch is praised for her formerly noxious scheme. This change of mind is a result of collective argumentation on the part of the customers, demonstrating that Ika Loch's authoritarian behavior towards them, which once ignored their personal desires, must be correct after all. The whole passage is couched in the formality of an argument, replete with terms from writings resembling the scientific method and such disciplines as psychology.

The passage starts with the sober opening statement (which is ironic, of course, from the reader's point of view) that "this change of opinion came about by a quite simple process." The argument unfolds as follows. Posit that the customers agreed that their wishes were not heeded by Ika Loch. Posit as a second proposition: the authoritarian attitude of Ika Loch was intolerable. Doubts eroded this initial proposition with the assumption that if Ika Loch was wrong about their desires in such an authoritarian manner, she must have had good reasons for her behavior and way of thinking. Conclusion "really already proven ab absurdo to be certain" – they are wrong and Ika Loch is right. This principal item of the fallacious reasoning engenders a set of secondary argumentations. The preceding assumption is proven by means of a formal fallacy. Proposition: Ika Loch is correct. Assumption: she cannot be wrong for this would imply a conscious wish for ruination. And madams who run brothels as business establishments do not want bankruptcy. The implied syllogism in this case is: madams are businessmen. Businessmen do not like bankruptcies. Therefore, this madam will not do anything to her clients which would incur a financial disaster.

A second thread of reasoning unravels from the main syllogism. It is based on the implied syllogism: madams are experts in sex. The client is not a madam. Therefore he is not an expert in sex. This line of reasoning is supported by the clients' recollection that psychoanalysis discovered their true sex life in the subconscious. Hence the real meaning of their sexual desires is made manifest when they are not conscious of them. If they wanted to know exactly what they desired, they should probe their dreams. But they had never controlled their dreams in order to establish exactly what their desires were. Therefore, they had no real notion of what they wanted. From this also follows that (since madams are sexual experts), Ika Loch knew what her customers wanted (and they knew they were wrong) and consequently must have studied psychoanalysis; ". . . one could not question the fact that she had mastered Freud from A to Z." This absurd reasoning satisfies everyone and clarifies everything for them. The customers were wrong, and Ika Loch correct in her assumptions. Ika Loch must be an expert in Freudian analysis. This fact now also explains her authoritarian behavior; it follows consequently from the feeling of superiority inherent in a disciple of Freud. The conclusion arrived at through this false reasoning in terms of the individual (Ika Loch) is extended to the genus; all madams should diligently study psychoanalysis.

But, interjects the impersonal narrator, this conclusion was a purely theoretical deduction. One needs energy or its surrogate, chance, to transform a theoretical conclusion into practice. The energy, in this instance chance, was supplied by the crime. And a practical application of the theoretical conclusion logically results in a booming business for Ika Loch's brothel. Then another series of logical conclusions follows, based on the foregoing argument. The demonstration proceeds *ad infinitum*. The reasoning and argumentation are relentless, and never discover the essential contrariety of the discourse. Fallacious syllogisms and reasoning are delivered in utter seriousness. The inversion of rationality becomes a cognitive reality. And the perpetrators go unmolested. Speciousness in this world does not imply ruination; error is truth. The obverse is a correlative to our world. In the grotesque world, grotesque reasoning is true. It is akin to the absurd world of *King Lear*, where the fool speaks of a man who "in pure kindness to his horse, buttered his hay." The important thing to remember is that this compassion is genuine, although it may seem ludicrous to the audience.

What is veracity to the customers of Ika Loch might to a reader seem semantic *spielerei*. Yet a careful examination of the style shows that the vehicle of this strange reasoning exercises its own inquest. There is a subtle artistry in the seemingly superficial sophism. Language, style and diction subtly undercut the positive conclusions of an essentially erroneous mode of reasoning. A negative became positive in the main syllogism outlined before. Now we can see how Van Ostaijen unobtrusively subverts this paradox until positive and negative cancel each other out, and we have arrived in a strange and fearful region where the obverse is everything and paradox the rule. Yet they in turn are again attacked and neutralized. The series of logical conclusions further and at the same time diminish the argument. Stripping the layers of an onion, we are left with nothing. The onion is no longer there, only a heap of layers remains which, together, went to make an onion. No kernel, no core. An onion is, so to speak, a mock of itself. It exists by virtue of a vegetable illusion as an onion. But essential "onionness" is never revealed. So with these tales. The layers of the argumentation, layers of language are stripped, revealed, codified, only to arrive at a void, a kernel of nothingness. Language is playing a conjurer's trick with antilanguage: silence and the void.

With this descriptive approximation of grotesque argumentation in mind, one may pursue the final result of the long series of positive arguments by Ika Loch's customers. The madam "remained authoritarian, only because she happened to be that way." That is to say, her authoritarianism had nothing to do with Freud and psychoanalysis. In fact, she was totally ignorant of both, and her entire behavior was simply based on error. The customers did preserve a measure of scepticism concerning her methods and her behavior, but this was negated by Ika Loch's dictatorial behavior as soon as they entered her establishment. So she was able to continue not to give her clients what they really desired, since they now realized that their wishes were superficial. The negatory basis of this argument is evident in the following conclusion, where the contradictory triumph is described in entirely negative terms: ". . . Ika Loch had managed to accomplish this masterpiece, to eliminate the essential desire, to suppress the sex drive in sex life; on the other hand, to force what was not even an existing desire as existing." The clientele is further ridiculed by the disclosure that some of them had no trouble adjusting to Ika Loch's regime, since they were already in a "succubine relationship" with women. The connotative annihilation is aided by the stylistic burlesque of a grave tone and state diction.

What Ika Loch dictates as pleasurable to her male charges does not correspond very favorably with their erstwhile notions about sexual pleasure. But they feel that the madam does what is humanly possible, and decide that what they used to enjoy were merely the illusions of puberty. The paragraph which records this strange justification is an example of a double negative supporting a positive conclusion. It is first of all negative because it was previously established that Ika Loch's system and behavior was based

on being intrinsically wrong. Language provides the second negation. In this single paragraph *not* is used six times in addition to *never, superficial, cancel out, illusion,* plus negative phrases and clauses. Stylistic negation anticipates a more general one when it becomes clear that Ika Loch has practically no understanding of sexual drives at all. A brief encounter behind a circus tent is the only experience she ever had. After this event, when still very young, she underwent a hysterectomy. Her lauded knowledge, therefore, is merely a professional interest, scarcely based on private experience. The logic which supports her professionalism is further negated by the additional information that this scientific procuress is myopic. From the sum of details, Ika Loch must fashion for herself an approximation of the charms of the woman she is matching with a customer whom, by implication, she can only see through optic induction. The author seems to be slyly suggesting that her authoritarianism was also a result of having to hide a physical shortcoming.

At this point the absurd argument seems to have come full circle. Ika Loch, the embodiment of cerebrality and logical reasoning, has finally been stripped of everything positive. Yet, she is highly successful and her establishment the pride of the city. The only conclusion one seems to be able to draw is that chance was really her master. "She had made unlucky chance into a chanceless norm." This formulation both annihilates the logic of the story, and at the same time, reinforces its absurd ratiocination; chance has been made an antithetical axiom. There is no end to this set of Chinese boxes.

Profuse ratiocination in these grotesques is an exaggeration, a caricature of the world's blatant faith in folly. The reality of the grotesques is a world turned topsy-turvy, and in order to represent it, excessive argumentation *ad absurdum* draws the reader's attention to this essential absurdity. Quite early in his career Van Ostaijen saw the powerful possibilities of exaggeration. Speaking of Van Gogh, he calls exaggeration indispensable in order to emphasize the essence of the artist's vision. He makes this principle axiomatic for modern art. "In order to represent reality *faithfully* [sic], one shall not put it on the canvas according to its specific proportions; but one shall exaggerate the preeminent characteristics, so that one can also attract attention to them." [9] Stylistically, deformation of syntax, ironic repetition and negating contradiction subtly exaggerate the absurdity of the grotesque's obsession with logical reasoning. The determination of these tales to argue the validity of their grotesqueness is exaggerated in order to criticize the world's blind devotion to positivistic logic. The method of discourse is not logical, but contiguous, and this only emphasizes its syllogistic nature.

Emphasis on contiguity of style prevents logical progression and preserves a strong feeling of suspension; the fictional vacuum thus created is in itself an exaggeration of the essential absurdity of the grotesque world. Metonymic art supports this axiomatic principle. A metonomy may be seen as a figure of speech which exaggerates an attribute of the thing meant. "Patriotism Incorporated" is a metonomy of chauvinism, Ika Loch of syllogistic reasoning, Scholem Weissbinder of a persecution complex, "The Lost House Key" of a syphilitic society. "The General" exaggerates man's innate desire for violence, "Mechtildis" is an hyperbole of the stereotyped prostitute with "a heart of gold," while the notary Telleke represents a caricature of the bourgeoisie. The individual tales are stylistic as well as thematic hyperboles of a grotesque world. In order to "faithfully represent" the reality of a world all topsy-turvy, Van Ostaijen exaggerates its "preeminent" absurdities to expose empirical reality's negative reversibility.

LANGUAGE AS A GAME OF DESTRUCTION

Finally, a quick glance at the diction of these tales. It is not surprising that in "Ika Loch's Brothel," a tale concerned with logic in an argumentative and semi-scientific fashion, the diction is abstract, formal and academic. An example of how prominent this kind of vocabulary can be is the following sentence, which consists almost entirely of abstract concepts. "That diagram, based on crude data, lead approximately to this practical result, that Ika Loch's success in her identifications barely exceeded the level of happy coincidence." This sentence also demonstrates another feature of this style and diction, the professed desire to be scientifically precise and neutral in observation. Hence the qualifying adjectives *crude* (*data*), *practical* (*result*), *happy* (*coincidence*); the modifying phrase (*that diagram*) *based on crude data*; the adverbs *approximately* (*lead*), *barely* (*exceeded*). This too is indicative of the rest of the tale.

But as in the case of the larger syntactical components of sentences and paragraphs, one may well ask whether precision has been achieved. A semblance is obtained through grammatical usage, but the sum of the qualitative adjuncts seldom achieves its ostensible purpose. The feigned precision is a counterfeit coin. Very often the modifiers are general and vague, and do not define the abstract nouns with which they are connected with great precision. The denotative quality of these modifiers is imprecise, while their connotative meaning is diverse and includes many possibilities. Hence the modifier's usual function of clarification is prevented by the skillful choice of diction. Taking the same sentence as example, one can see that modifiers such as *crude* (*data*), *approximately* (*lead*), *barely* (*exceeded*), *happy* (*coincidence*) negate or neutralize in varying degrees their grammatical assignations. Language is constantly waging guerilla warfare against intended sense and content. Actually, the usages from the exact and other sciences are rather helpless in this nullifying discourse. The grotesque discourse is a lecture written on palimpsest.

A passage which attempts, with the aid of scientific terminology, to define Ika Loch's conception of the desires of the amorphous mass of men between twenty-five and forty-five eludes its purpose and ultimately negates precision and definition. One is impressed, at first, by the erudition of the discourse. But then one quickly notes semantic diffusion, and one begins to ask what precisely are "psycho-cerebral-value-amalgams"? Mathematical equations are of little help either. The customers, when they are in the company of the women appointed to them by the madam, try to establish the nature of their sexual drives by means of the following equation: "... given the partner determined by Ika Loch, X, find the value of Z. Ika Loch's authority guaranteed that the relation X–Z was not based on a mistake, not even on an *erreur sentimentale*." Which is both true and false since, as was pointed out previously, Ika Loch's system and behavior is based on error and ignorance of facts, but also on cerebrality.

The formal tone is also maintained through deliberately chosen antiquated diction. The relative pronoun *dewelke* ("who" or "which"), often used in these tales, is formal and antiquarian usage. It is very seldom used in modern Dutch (*die* being the correct and common usage), and it gives a deliberately stilted effect. *Kornuiten* ("companions") is also formal usage, though it often contains a derogatory implication. *Ongekunsteld* is a formal synonym for "simple" or "natural." *Euvel nemen* ("to take fault") is in the same category of stilted usage. These are some examples from the very first paragraph of the tale. The remainder is equally riddled with formal, dated, or antiquated usage in order to obtain a tone of formality.

This calculated use of language for specific effects takes another form in what is generally known as "wordplay." There are rimes in prose sentences, and such purposely misused words as *krasse systematiek* ("sprightly systematization"). *Kras* is an adjective used to indicate sprightliness or a certain element of youthfulness in an elderly person; e.g., *hij is een krasse man*. It may also be applied to concepts, though this usage is dated, and generally only found in set phrases. In this context, it is something of a malapropism, yet it manages at the same time to connote a negative reflection on Ika Loch's system. A definite malapropism is the following admonition by Ika Loch to one of her girls, Anais. "Ik verzoek je daarop acht te geven, zodat ik je deze les niet meer heb te spellen." The correct idiom is *iemand de les lezen*. Ika Loch's stilted reprimand to Anais becomes ridiculous with this idiomatic mistake. Instances of such word-play are countless in the grotesques, and can be the basis even for an entire story, such as "The Marvelous Novel." Van Ostaijen delights, so to speak, in constantly taking language and meaning for a ride.

One must conclude that diction is also used as a double-edged sword. It is usually formal, abstract and technical, to fit the argumentative and dis-cursive tone of the tale. Yet, as in the case of syntactical elements, the very usage which seemingly supports the narrative framework really destroys it. Sly, erosive, working by innuendo, the diction works counter to what is expected from it. Language will not be harnessed under the yoke of a scientific method. Language has its own life, and has a disconcerting capacity to laugh at that which it upholds. Ultimately, nothing is certain. These ponderous and porous discourses remind one of lectures delivered by the Mad Hatter.

LUDIC LANGUAGE

From the foregoing discussion one can infer certain stylistic aspects of the grotesque in general, and of these tales in particular. This is neither a style of romantic expansiveness, nor of naturalistic documentation, but an au-thentic modern rhetoric. The author is objective to the point of anonimity. Like an indifferent god he watches the fictional events unfold with what Salomon Friedlaender called "schöpferische Indifferenz." This creative indifference allows a peculiar parataxis of style and content; it exploits an equality which lavishes the same attention on the mundane as on the ab-stract concept. When the trivial and the sublime change places there is no discernible upheaval in the conceptual hierarchy; all things are equal in this language. What words denote to our preconceptions is immaterial to the language of the grotesque. Whatever connotations we register and use for judgment are entirely our affair and, if possible, language will try its best to subvert these, too, through ambiguous modifications. The "Affektlosig-keit" (Kayser) of this democratic objectivity has a disturbing influence on the reader. There is no emotional perspective. The critical attitude extracted from the tale „Ika Loch's Brothel" was one of stylistic innuendo.

Language will perpetrate anything, even the seemingly impossible. Language is independent and autonomous. It is content and expression. In our literate world language usurps the throne of reason and rules tyrannic-ally, destroying our naive trust in its veracity. One way of representing its arbitrary nature is the oscillation from one extreme to another, for example, excessively long, formal discourses counterpointed by an equivocal brief concluding sentence, which destroys our traditional view of language's reasonable progression from one established certainty to another. Baudelaire described this type of language and its intent very well: ". . . la phrase poétique peut imiter (et par là elle touche à l'art et à la science mathématique) la ligne horizontale, la ligne droite ascendante, la ligne droite descendante; qu'elle peut monter à pic vers le ciel, sans essoufflement, ou descendre perpendiculairement vers l'enfer avec la vélocité de toute pesanteur; qu'elle peut suivre la spirale, décrire la parabole, ou le zigzag figurant une série d'angles superposés . . ."[10] This destruction of norms is perpetrated by means of a mocking rhetoric, a perverse resemblance to rational discourse.

Language, like a devout medieval scholastic, gravely widens the division between *ens reale* and *ens rationis*. It places us in a world of *entia rationis* or conceptual entities, which crush reality under the artifice of language. It will exhibit observable properties, but leaves existence in the stockroom. The positivism of the modern world, which has put so much trust in language that it has sacrificed reality to semantics on many occasions, now sees itself burlesqued by the medium of its triumph. Language turns against its master; it inverts hypotheses and axiomatic truths, makes logical positivism seem a cruel joke. Using the techniques which elected it into legislative office – the techniques of reason, conceptual thinking, intellect and artifice – it now proceeds with acquired throughness to undo what it was taught to create. But beneath the stylistics, beneath the artifice, a world awry goes on living. The stylized formality is clear from the use of rhetorical figures as they were outlined above. One noted how formal principles energetically built structures in their own image, and how these absolute formal principles were subverted. In this world of polarity and paradox, construction is destruction: *Bau ist Abbau*. Reason has become the stone of Sisyphus.

A world which creates havoc with everyday reality through its most trusted medium (language), must have its humorous aspects. There is the verbal humor of wordplay, conscious misapplication of correct usage, syntactical inversion and deformations. Humor is created by disregarding facts, normality, rationality and by a ludicrous transformation of traditional certainties. But this humor seldom arouses laughter which lasts as a form of release. The sardonic amusement of these tales creates an apprehensive shudder. Perhaps all one can say is that Van Ostaijen is amused by the object of his observation, but is not amusing in his expression of the notation of that object. If we laugh in these tales, we are not relieved. The objectivity which encompasses the ludicrous as well as the sublime does not precipitate merriment. It is a reflective humor; seriousness is being assaulted and played with. But this does not imply hearty belly-laughs either. The very inclusion of the principle of distortion in a style which reveals an essentially foolish world has an unsettling effect.

The employment of comic techniques (inversion, contrast, repetition, distortion) in such a formal style presupposes humor. And one does find various manifestations of that Protean entity in these tales: satire, irony, burlesque. But one must insist on the paradox that, in most cases, the humor is not funny. There are comic elements in the style and in the tales as a whole. But the net result is a constriction, a foreboding, a presentiment of disaster. It appears from the evidence of the style that this elusive and perplexing concept of humor enters the discussion as a result of the principle of distortion, which is basic to the style. Almost by reflex one assumes that distortion implies a comic mode. But distortion is essentially a negative process. A look through the bifocals of atrophy and hypertrophy evokes laughter as the initial reaction to their distortion. But this laughter is soon strangled by fear. Again the author has lead his reader skillfully into a trap. Recognizing certain elements which, traditionally, will entertain an audience, the reader followed the author's inducements to find the tables turned. Entertainment has become deadly serious and has turned around to laugh at its audience. This is the effect Van Ostaijen desires in his grotesques as he clearly illustrated in "Intermezzo." With this brief consideration of the perplexing role of humor an impasse seems to have been reached. But a discussion of this enigmatic quality points slyly to its correlative: the element of play.

The tales' stylistic elements all point to a playful atmosphere. In the grotesques Van Ostaijen is indulging his *facultas ludendi*. With the concept of a *facultas ludendi* one has come perhaps closest to a classification of the various elements under discussion. Language seems to be playing a cat and mouse game with reality. It is relentless; there is no such thing as an altruistic cat. The rhetorical devices combine into an ironic playing with stylistic techniques; the entire verbal structure is an anti-world. Nothing resembles quotidian reality (though it was used as the foundation) once this subtle process of demolition is accomplished upon what appeared to be normality. Logic is only a mockery of itself; reason refutes itself; paradox is the kernel of the grotesque world. Nothing is sacred. An essentially foolish world cannot be depicted in an essentially serious fashion. But one can toy with it, mock it, play a game with its absurdity, if only to maintain control over one's sense of horror.

The Dutch scholar Huizinga in his well-known book *Homo Ludens* (Haarlem, 1958) describes the play element in our culture in terms relevant to the grotesque. A game is irrational, yet spiritual; it is "supralogical." Language is a play element par excellence. A game can be very serious and cerebral; is not necessarily silly or foolish, and for the participants it is not comical at all. Playing is an autonomous manifestation not subjected to ordinary life. It demands absolute freedom for itself, and within this autonomy, creates its own time and laws. The basic characteristics of the game, according to Huizinga, are repetition, contrast and contradiction; yet a game creates an order which, though of its own making, is nevertheless absolute. As the discussion of the style implied, a similar sense of order can be found in these tales. The preponderance of negative qualities does not exclude the possibility of order. There is method in madness; order is limited by disorder. A game has a tension created by a presentiment of uncertainty, of chance. One cannot be sure of anything in a game. Yet this element of qualified uncertainty has a palpable fascination. Perhaps this goes to explain the unsettling fascination which these tales have, despite their attempt to be contrary to everything we deem normal. Within the ramifications of the game, the laws and customs of ordinary life have been terminated and are no longer valid. In a sense the game is a diversion for outlaws from reality. Knackfuss, the rogue of "The Gang of the Trunk," is well aware of this fact when he is about to operate on the unfortunate Marquis de Mirlitonare. "From the point of view of a natural morality, you have richly deserved this operation. What could be more natural than that I profit from this morality to carry on my business, since I am an outlaw. I welcome any morality." (III, 81) There is a suspension of reality which shrouds the game with an air of mystery. The enigmatic quality only enhances its attractiveness. Finally, the desire to shed normality finds expression in an element of exaggeration in the game.

Huizinga's descriptive analysis of the play element in our culture parallels the characteristics of Van Ostaijen's prose style. It also sheds some light on the difficult problem of the brand of humor these tales exhibit. To an outsider, i.e. one firmly planted in reality, a game with its own rules and techniques can seem ludicrous and comical. However, within the sharply defined context of the game itself, they are perfectly plausible, natural and serious. What in these tales seems to be capricious toying is in fact a game with the absurd. In "Patriotism Incorporated," Wybau, the other true outlaw of these tales besides Knackfuss, has managed to perform a feat of mass-suggestion. The people of Fochany are convinced that the landmark of their capital, the "Neiffeltower," has been stolen by the enemy. They are broadcasting this heinous deed to the world from the radio station on top of the tower. Wybau is modest about his achievement. "It's nothing, a game, but intellect is nothing but a game." (III, 52) "The General" from Peru sees the games of children as the archetype of true warfare. "No generally important children's game but it evolves from the lust for war." (III, 338) Such games are not funny. Salomon Friedlaender the German philosopher and writer of grotesques, summarizes the grotesque's mode of playing quite succinctly. "Der Irrtum ist eine so reale Macht wie die Wahrheit." [11]

One final problem remains. How does one classify a style which is bent on expressing itself out of existence? Van Ostaijen made his own attempt in his hybrid tale (part essay, part monologue) "Between Fire and Water." In this work of prose Van Ostaijen tries to describe the mental state between sleeping and being awake. The discussion never states how this experience can be defined with real precision. But in the course of attempting to do so, he distinguishes between "arabesque" and "dream." What kind of thinking is enclosed in this state between not-being-quite awake and not-quite-dreaming? He gives the following proportional scale. If one gives concrete thought the number 1 and dreaming the number 4, then one may see arabesque-thinking as 2 and the state of suspension between sleep and consciousness as number 3; i.e., the arabesque is an intermediary state between thinking and dreaming. The arabesque is sequential, but is a series of transitions dependent upon "causal fortuity and fortuitous causality." It is not a history, but superficial and ornamental. The dream, however, is closer to concrete thought. Like concrete thought it also insists on a systematic history. The arabesque takes no stand at all in relation to concrete thinking, while the dream, on the contrary, is hostile to it. The dream is an unconscious reaction to normative thought: ". . . the dream is living out the subconscious in such a grotesque manner that it becomes a critique of normal thinking." (III, 22) The dream has order and legislates its own laws, though in a fashion hostile to conscious thought. "I say, therefore, that the dream has a system which is exactly contrary to conscious existence, the episode in the dream is epistemologically absurd because it strives to be epistemologically correct in conscious thought." (III, 23)

Having described both the arabesque and the dream in terms of thought – both being contrary to conscious, concrete thinking – Van Ostaijen then tries to describe the particular mode of thought which he is experiencing. It is not an arabesque, because his thinking is not as clear as an arabesque. Nor is it like dream-thought, because things happen sequentially, ". . . and the periods of this sequence are mostly cut off by perceptions of the outside world." The closest he can get to describing it is by calling it a "veiled arabesque." The style of these tales obviously has qualities of both these modes of thought as they are described by Van Ostaijen, though it seems generally closer to his description of dream-thought. Yet its sequentiality and abstraction is akin to the arabesque. Instead of calling it a "veiled arabesque," it would perhaps be more appropriate, within the context of his definition, to describe it with the phrase – this style is like dream-thought expressed by means of an arabesque.

Nevertheless, discussions of the grotesque style which circle around terminology such as *dream*, *arabesque*, or *nonsense* must remain circuitous. Roger Shattuck, for example, in trying to define the style of modern writing and painting, makes use of *nonsense* and *dream*, assigning the former a rigorous logic all its own through an "absolute control over its objects," while the latter thrives on disorganization, on "association and disorder." He must immediately admit, however, that in many cases of individual authors and artists the distinction does not hold, and that they "produced works which cross and recross the fine line between highly suggestive dream sequence and utterly cool, playful nonsense." [12] The discussion of Van Ostaijen's narrative essay showed that he reversed Shattuck's distinction. Van Ostaijen contends that the dream has a rigorous logic all its own, and legislates the element of fortuitousness to what he calls the "arabesque," the counterpart of Shattuck's "nonsense."

What then do all these features add up to? Perhaps a descriptive summation of the style of the grotesques as a unit might formulate a working hypothesis for the form of these modern narrative artifices. Keeping its principal features of cerebrality, contradiction, inversion, and absurdity in mind, one might call a grotesque by Van Ostaijen a paralogical structure. Paralogism comes from the Greek παραλογίζεθαι, meaning "to reason falsely," stressing its use as an unconscious act; i.e., as opposed to sophism. One could however reverse this, stating that a highly conscious artist can construct a paralogical structure which gives the impression of having been an act of the unconscious, a sophisticated paralogism. In his poetry, Van Ostaijen opted for the most concentrated form of lyricism, "the shortest possible distance between vision and expression," to reach the profundity of "l'aperception première." The lengthy, circular paralogistic amblings of the grotesques are the exact obverse of his "clenched lyricism." The grotesques do not penetrate through empirical reality, but expose its negative reversibility.

These are different aims but, in a sense, both are antimaterialistic modes of metonymic expression. The grotesques negate or discard many conventional narrative devices: there is reduction of characterization, dramatic elements, transitional devices. Style and content gradually merge to form a *gegenstandslose Kunst*, which becomes an independent, autonomous creation. Such a development occurs also in metonymic art, according to Roman Jakobson's theory. "In diesem Sinne bekunden die metonymische Verbindungen ... einen beharrlichen Hang zur Gegenstandslosigkeit, der auch die anderen Kunstformen der nämlichen Epoche kennzeichnet. Die geschaffene Verbindung wird an und für sich zum Gegenstand." Thus these tales are not mere decorative ornamentations. With what are essentially anarrative methods, they are intended to *mean* something, they are intended to formulate antithetically a world of the absurd. Gradually the grotesques develop into stylistic variations on a single theme. "The Gang of the Trunk" has more conventional narrative devices than, for example, "The General," which almost exclusively deals with the paralogical exposition of an incongruous conception of warfare. But the problem is how to reconcile the logical, almost mathematical elements of these tales with the absurdity they intend to disclose. Ratiocination is a parody of chaos; the sense of the complete veracity one gets from these discourses mocks their absurd premise. In fact, the stern authority of the delivery enhances a feeling of presentiment.

This bizarre relationship between order and chaos is not only indigenous to modern artistic movements, but finds a precedent, for example, in sixteenth century mannerism. G. R. Hocke in *Die Welt als Labyrinth* aptly formulates this curious confrontation across the ages between, let us say, Cubism and Leonardo da Vinci.

Man fängt die sich ins Ungegenständliche verflüchtigten Bildinhalte mit Netzen geometrischer Formen wieder ein. Theodor Heuss spricht daher mit recht von einer "akzentuierten Geometrik" als "Rettung aus dem Chaos der Zeit." Damit ergibt sich eine der ersten typischen manieristischen Reaktionen auf Manierismen, die so bezeichnend für unsere Gegenwart, für unsere verschiedenen "Schulen" und "Gruppen" sind für ihre leidenschaftlichen Rivalitäten; einige sind sie nur in ihrem ebenso passionierten Anti-Klassizismus und Anti-Naturalismus. Schon im 16. Jahrhundert soll die labyrinthische "Welt sonder Ende" wieder begrenzt werden, durch eine brutale Hervorhebung elementarer geometrischer Formstrukturen im Raume, in den Dingen, in der menschlichen Gestalt. Im 16. Jahrhundert wird der Kubismus geboren.

Following Hocke's exploration of manneristic style, some useful descriptive notions can be applied to the style of Van Ostaijen's grotesques.

Hocke speaks primarily in pictorial terms which, however, do not prevent their application to Van Ostaijen's prose style. Anyone acquainted with his life and work will remember the close association, which was at times almost a symbiosis, of the pictorial arts and his prose and poetry. In fact, the gradual elimination of narrative conventions culminates in a series of short prosepieces which approximate abstract word-paintings, to be discussed separately. They are the final phase of the prose style of the grotesques. As present and subsequent discussions should indicate, Paul Rodenko was quite correct in calling Van Ostaijen the "Mondriaan of narrative prose." [13]

Given the theme of a world out of joint, everything can be transformed in terms of this negative proposition. In this sense, mindful of Jakobson's theory, one could call the grotesques abstract metonymies of an absolute incongruity. Negativity is expressed by contiguous components and structures. As in the poetry, the cumulative effect of isolated, perhaps unalterable components *combine* into an organic structure. That which cannot be expressed, such as the concept nil, might not be comprehended discursively, but can be represented by images. Hence, metonymies may be seen as an urge for abstraction, to express what is discursively inexpressible. So-called "classical grotesques" transform, exaggerate, transfer disparate elements of life; forms from flora and fauna are commingled with human forms; the inorganic is made organic; inanimate is suddenly animate. This is just one stage of abstracting, of expressing the inexpressible. Hocke calls such artistic efforts in painting or literature a *Para-Rhetorik*.

This related series of terms, from the general concept of a paralogic through reciprocal forms such as a para-rethoric and contiguous metonymies, share formal deviation, share a peculiar shift in focus. Thus, one could finally call the grotesques an art of anamorphosis, from ἀνά and μορφή meaning "form," the Aristotelian determinant of matter. The *Oxford English Dictionary* provides the following very applicable definition of the grotesques in terms of the concept anamorphosis. *Anamorphosis* is "a distorted projection or drawing of anything, which, when viewed from a particular point, or by reflection from a suitable mirror, appears regular and properly proportioned; a deformation."

The grotesques are distortions of reality and of traditional narrative norms, yet their impact is one of veracity, order and proportion. A distortion has become regularity, incongruity congruous, absurdity everyday reality. Through an optical illusion of narrative fiction, the reader has come to believe in a world of absurdity. With consummate skill far from alleged ineptness, Van Ostaijen has managed to make the reader realize, through a process of delayed reaction, the persuasive and pervasive power of the grotesque world. It is a world where, as Shakespeare saw,

> reason can revolt
> Without perdition, and loss assume all reason
> Without revolt.

THE FINAL PHASE; VAN OSTAIJEN'S LYRICAL PROSE AS A LANGUAGE OF PERCEPTION

The ten prose pieces which are discussed in this chapter have, with one exception, been treated only in a cursory fashion.[1] Scant critical examination of these difficult pieces has usually offered little more illuminating than an abstract adverb. Perhaps one reason for this respectful neglect might be their apparent cryptic and impenetrable quality. The present effort attempts to discuss these pieces within a coherent framework of theoretical correlatives, thereby seeking to give access to, but not explain away, their characteristic enigmatic quality. Theoretical correlations which form the foundation of the discussion are the continental philosophy of phenomenology, Roman Jakobson's previously mentioned theory of metonymic writing and, with three specific pieces in mind, Kandinsky's theory of art.

The texts are the following two collections and two separate pieces. *Four Short Tales* (*Vier korte vertellingen*, III, 213–219) include "Aquarelle" ("Aquarel," 215), "Anais" (216–217), "Convictions" ("Overtuigingen," 218) and "Curious Attack" ("Merkwaardige aanval," 219–220). Their date of composition is unknown; their first date of publication was in 1924. Of these four, "Aquarelle" and "Curious Attack" will be discussed in terms of Kandinsky's theory of art; "Anais" is used to draw a parallel interpretation, while "Convictions" remains unmentioned, since it is clearly of the genre of the longer grotesques, discussed previously. "The Sirens" ("De Sirenen," 244–245) is usually published as part of the collection *Zoo for Children of Our Time* (*Diergaarde voor Kinderen van Nu*, 231–246), a series of grotesque *jeux d'esprit* or *jeux des mots*. However, "The Sirens" exhibits a somewhat different spirit, seems more attuned to the prose-poems under discussion here, showing a greater sensitivity and feeling for nuances of a more transcendental kind than the other pieces in the collection.[2] "The Sirens" is discussed in the present chapter in conjunction with a brief excursion into the vast domain of "Kafkaiana," in order to establish Van

Ostaijen, with the exception of some Czech translations, as one of the very first translators of this Czech/German writer.

Four Prose Pieces (*Vier proza's*, 247–253) contain "Little forest" ("Het Bosje," 249), "Nicolas" (250–251), "Lines" ("Lijnen," 252) and "O Thou, My Splendid Solitude" ("O gij, mijn schone eenzaamheid," 253). There is some evidence that they were written during 1927 and first published in 1928.[3] Phenomenology and metonymic art provide the frame of reference to clarify some of the mystery of content and composition these pieces might have for casual readers. "Obsequies" ("De Uitvaart," 398) is considered to be of the same type as these *Four Prose Pieces*.[4] The bibliographical evidence Borgers supplies for this posthumously published piece argues just as well for its having been written in 1927 as in 1926. Leaving the problem of dating aside, "Obsequies" belongs thematically most definitely to the *Four Prose Pieces*.

The present chapter is intended not only to round off a relatively complete study of Van Ostaijen's creative efforts in prose, but also to present for the first time a detailed investigation of these pieces as a relative unity. Furthermore, these works do have a link which connects them with the genre of the major grotesques. As poetic prose *Dichtungen* of metonymic art they refer back, stylistically, to the grotesques discussed previously. While the grotesques, in broad outlines, were classified as examples of Jakobson's metonymic art, these nine *poëmata* (as Van Ostaijen called the kindred prose pieces by Kafka which he translated in 1924) are specific and condensed examples of this type of poetic discourse.

METONYMIC ART: ROMAN JAKOBSON AND PAUL VAN OSTAIJEN

The main link between the grotesques and the prose pieces discussed in this chapter is metonymic art. As was pointed out previously, Van Ostaijen's grotesques may be classified under Roman Jakobson's heading of metonymic art, a form of writing in which development is by contiguity, with metonymy as its most condensed expression. Jakobson's "bipolar structure of language," i.e. either metaphoric or metonymic, has the convenience of clarity, though still allowing a range of overlapping situations between the two poles.[5] Van Ostaijen's art, in both poetry and prose, is generally speaking most assuredly a metonymic art form. Jakobson calls poetry predominantly metaphoric and prose essentially a metonymic form of artistic expression, but we have in Van Ostaijen a case where the poetry as well as the prose is strongly metonymic. It is a revealing coincidence that Jakobson calls Cubism "manifestly metonymically oriented,"[6] while Van Ostaijen remained throughout his career primarily interested in cubistic art. At this point only a few salient aspects of Jakobson's metonymic art, as he studied it in Pasternak's prose, juxtaposed to theoretical statements by Van Ostaijen, must suffice to establish a similarity between the linguist's theory and the Flemish author's creative work as well as theory.

The major characteristic of metonymic art is development by contiguity. Jakobson differentiates between the metaphor's exploration of similarity, real or irreal, and metonymy's employment of contiguity. Van Ostaijen calls his organic lyricism a "series" (IV, 120) of phenomena elicited from "various zones of experience set side by side." (IV, 129) Van Ostaijen most clearly formulates Jakobson's contiguity in a passage already quoted before: "The various associatively connected realities lie *next to each other.*" "The theme of the poem is here, so to speak, the agreed upon subject; all the associations are the various predicates, laid according to their value next to each other, which, as elements, gradually build up this subject from themselves." (IV, 245) Van Ostaijen is adamantly opposed to metaphoric poetry. "In place of the metaphor, we posit association. It happens that the entire poem is but one claim of associatively connected realities ... All comparative tendencies, however, are alien to association. Why do we choose association? Because it is more positive; that which is associated does not function here any longer as explaining or clarifying the primary element." (IV, 130) Obviously, Van Ostaijen's "association" is Jakobson's "contiguity."

Jakobson clearly indicates that metonymic art creates its own autonomous existence. For the Russian poet Chlebnikov, his created world is so constructed that ". . . ihm jedes Zeichen, jedes geschaffene Wort mit einer vollen selbständigen Realität ausgestattet ist und die Frage nach seinem Bezug zu irgend einem aussenliegenden Gegenstand, ja die Frage der Existenz eines solchen Gegenstandes wird vollkommen überflüssig." "Die geschaffene Verbindung wird an und für sich zum Gegenstand." In Van Ostaijen's theory of organic lyricism, the hegemony of the poem itself, corresponds to this autonomy created by metonymic art. "Organic prosody: sentences or word-series perfect in themselves, a logical development from the premise and a conclusion which motivates in a lyrico-logical manner the positing of the premise." (IV, 322) For Van Ostaijen, the poet seeks primarily" . . . une indépendance formelle des organes qui, par après, constitueront l'ensemble organique du poème ... Seule me satisfait une construction lyrique formée de parties d'un contour précis et qui ne doivent pas emprunter leur force et leur beauté à l'ensemble."[7] Jakobson says that "eine beliebige Kontiguität kann als kausale Reihe aufgefasst werden"; Van

Ostaijen shares the same idea when he describes the sequence of a poem as having "only a very accidental phenomenal-causal relationship, but the lyrico-causal on the other hand has a clarity which leaves nothing to be desired." (IV, 291) Again, when Jakobson speaks of a "metonymische Wahlverwandtschaft" between images, Van Ostaijen demands a search for "les affinités électives des mots." [8]

Pasternak's creative prose is described by Jakobson as "ein Reich zu selbständigem Leben erweckter Metonymien," a description quite applicable to Van Ostaijen's later poetry and the poëmata under discussion. Repeatedly Jakobson stresses the independence of the objects created by metonymic art. "Die Äusserung des Gegenstandes nimmt auf sich seine Funktion ... Die Abstraktion wird zu selbständigen Handlungen befähigt, und diese Handlungen werden wiederum vergegenständlicht." This self-sufficiency of the created work of metonymic art corresponds to Van Ostaijen's notion of aseity. "What I want ... to make clear is that both in organic-expressionistic poetry and in organic-expressionistic painting there is a strive for formal aseity, for a construction consisting of the weighing against each other of parts in themselves already perfect, an aseity which in its nature remains close to the primary psychic or imaginative experience of the event ..." (IV, 241) The prose-pieces discussed her are more concise realizations of Van Ostaijen's poetic theory than the longer tales. They are therefore also much clearer examples of metonymic art, though one must always remember that the general style of the grotesques is decidedly a metonymic one. The grotesques, the poëmata and the lyrics are controlled by what Jakobson calls a "Berührungsassoziation," and use metonymic art's anthropomorphic techniques and synecdochic details as well as the various possibilities of contiguity and metonymy outlined in Jakobson's essay on Pasternak. Van Ostaijen's work belongs to Jakobson's "Reich zu selbtständigem Leben erweckter Metonymien."

Towards the end of his essay, Jakobson hints at an argument that metonymic art could be associated with phenomeonolgy. Linking Pasternak's metonymic art to cubistic painting, he accentuates one particular criterion which, in effect, sums up the phenomenological mode of knowing: ". . . die gegenseitige Durchdringung der Gegenstände (die Realisierung der Metonymie im eigentlichen Sinne). . ." A little later he again mentions a Weltanschauung which may be interpreted as phenomenological, and is presently applied by the nouveau-romanciers in France. "Zeige uns deine Umgebung, und ich sage dir, wer du bist ... die Handlung ist durch Topographie ersetzt." Finally, metonymic art moves "zur äussersten Verselbständigung des Zeichens vom Gegenstand," and Jakobson warns against biographical or ideological misrepresentations of this new form of art, but advices to link it rather to "der Hang der Philosophie zur Gegenständlich keit."

PHENOMENOLOGY: THE ADVENTURE OF CONSCIOUSNESS

This "Hang der Philosophie zur Gegenständlichkeit" was formulated as phenomenology during the first quarter of this century, and is still in a process of development in Germany and France.[9] Primarily a continental reformulation of reason (as opposed to Anglo-American schools of empiricism), its main German figures are Edmund Husserl and Martin Heidegger, while in France Jean-Paul Sartre and Maurice Merleau-Ponty have developed its Gallic branch. What follows is obviously not meant as an exhaustive treatment of such a complex philosophical revolution. A brief outline merely describes phenomenology's general intention and its modification in three major figures: Husserl, Heidegger and Merleau-Ponty. Its relevance to Van Ostaijen's work should become clear, and provide a basis for discussing these prose pieces as poetic crystallization of phenomenological ontology.

The Swiss philosopher Pierre Thévenaz summarizes the general intentions and aims of phenomenology as combining "the most radical break with our ordinary and natural attitude vis-à-vis the world (in this sense, it is an ascesis of the mind) with the deepening or the consecration of this original attitude (in this sense, it is respect for the real and engagement in the world). Consciousness takes its distance with regard to things; it gives itself complete freedom in respect to them, but one realizes at once that this is in order to be more faithful to our essential insertion in the world." Though it is very methodical in its investigations of the world and man's perception of it (the rigorousness of Husserl for example), phenomenology, however, is more of "an adventure of consciousness ... than a system of the world or a *Weltanschauung*." But this philosophy prides itself on its extreme objectivism in the search for essences, "of restoring the most originary real in all its meaning." Phenomenology in general is "description, but it is more than that: it is radical searching for foundations, transcendentalism. It presents itself as method, and yet it implies a complete view of the world. It is a disclosure of phenomena, but at the same time it is a return to the self or to the subject. It aims at essences, and it ends up in existence. It puts in parentheses the factual and the psychological datum, and yet it finally restores the lived world." (Thévenaz, 90–91)

This new and radical search in continental philosophy for the authenticity of phenomena of our world is echoed in modern criticism by the insistence

on the autonomy of the work of art itself. Monroe C. Beardsley has briefly
described this aesthetic revolution in criticism from Russian "Formalism"
to American "New Criticism." [10] Phenomenology champions the independence of the essence of the phenomenon, while in the new developments
of aesthetics, a successful battle has been fought to establish the hegemony
of the work of art. Both share a strong desire for objectivity (in aesthetics
the separation of the author from his work) and the autonomous existence
of the phenomenon (be it a poem or a tree). Though only critical correlatives, it is, nevertheless, amazing to notice how closely Van Ostaijen's
theory adheres to this new perspective shared by both philosophy and
aesthetics. For example, it has been mentioned already in connection with
the grotesques, that Van Ostaijen insisted on a maintenance of distance by
the artist of the grotesque, a distance which "never joins in the mad dance
of things." (IV, 129) Objectivity and distance are central to Van Ostaijen's
theory of art. "Hence I see a very modern, unpathetic, impersonally heroic
attitude." (IV, 179) A variation of this theoretical kernel is Van Ostaijen's
demand for disindividualization, which was also mentioned before. He sees
it as a "flight from the empirical" (just as phenomenology is in opposition
to empiricism), and finds that "this striving for disindividualization is the
most important feature of what I would like to call modern art." (IV, 126)

Van Ostaijen continues to add to the series of overlapping concepts
pertaining to this modern revolt against empiricism and naturalism with
his concept of exteriorization. Very close to phenomenological "reduction,"
Van Ostaijen's *l'extériorisation* will be discussed a little further on in connection with Husserl's *Einklammerung*. Just as the phenomenologist preserves the autonomy of the phenomenon, and the New Critic insists "that
a literary work should be read as an organic whole, self-existing and self-
sufficient, in all its complexity and unity," [11] Van Ostaijen argued consistently for the independent "organism" of the poem. In a speech of 1925,
he states that in poetry "je recherche d'abord une indépendence formelle
des organes qui, par après, constitueront l'ensemble organique du poème." [12]

This separation of author and work – so essential in grotesque art where
the artist does not want to be tainted by the world of absolute *verkeerdheid*
he is depicting – this disindividualization and the organic independence of
the poem, are constantly recurring *leitmotivs* in Van Ostaijen's critical
essays. If a poem may be seen as a Husserlian phenomenon and as New
Criticism's "organic whole," the similarity between them and Van Ostaijen
is striking. "Not the poet, but lyricism is its own end. I do not want poems
where the human aspect is open and avowed. I want a poem that is a
poem and that gives deliverance only through its almost imperceptible

vibrations . . ." (IV, 360) The following remarks by Van Ostaijen could have been quoted by a New Critic. "I strive for the complete poverty of the subject, so that the mind is not distracted by anything secondary, by anything which is not pure lyricism, and only because within this poverty my lyricism, a plant which needs sand and not clay, can develop itself . . . The most common rhetorician and the smallest high school boy have more to tell than I do. I want only my lyricism. Lyricism is a germ which has been little studied up till now." (IV, 321) In his reiterated insistence on the organic autonomy of the poem, on the aseity of words and lyrical components, on the anonymity of the author in relation to his work, Van Ostaijen defended and practiced the demands of a modern aesthetic theory which in turn is so closely associated with the philosophical development of phenomenology.

Husserl: "zu den Sachen selbst"

Edmund Husserl, the founder of phenomenology, in trying to find a third possibility between realism and idealism, admonished philosophy to turn to the object, to turn "zu den Sachen selbst." Husserl wanted to "see what it is that is really given in experience when we scrutinize it without any obscuring and empty preconceptions." [13] Even at this point we find some echoes of this Husserlian notion in Van Ostaijen. In his early essay, "Expressionism in Flanders," he notes that Expressionism has a reverence for the object as *Idee an sich*. (IV, 11–12) Phenomenology as philosophy became more descriptive than dialectical, finding its present terminus in Heidegger's re-evaluation of some of the most basic philosophical terminology, which had been traditionally accepted as constants. The two key terms of Husserl's inquiry are consciousness and phenomenon; i.e., the world or its various phenomena. Consciousness is *weltlich*, a "concrete (non-empirical) datum." [14] "The object is not *constructed* by this consciousness; it gives itself to the view of this consciousness." [15] This is what Husserl called the *Selbstgebung* of the object.

The trancendentalism of Husserl results from his famous "bracketing" of the world or phenomenological "reduction." "What is 'reduced' is . . . the world, the ensemble of all the empirical, rational, and even scientific judgments that we make about the world . . ." Such a reduction does not eliminate the world; its purpose is to "bring to light this essential intentional contact between consciousness and the world, a relationship which in the natural attitude remains veiled." [16] Husserl's famous *Einklammerung* is, according to Monroe Beardsley, one important link between phenomenology and the method and intention of modern "objectivist" aesthetics. Van Ostaijen again provides remarkable parallels. Discussing a canvas by Heinrich Campendonck, Van Ostaijen speaks of independent pictorial objects (a table, a pipe) and of himself as an objective "director" of these pictorial "characters." But that I of Van Ostaijen the observer is bracketed to permit the painting's fully independent existence: "le régisseur serait ce moi que l'on devrait déterminer négativement et positivement par la parenthèse . . ." (IV, 135) For Van Ostaijen, empirical knowledge of objects is irrelevant and obstructs the creative unity of the lyrical organism. He would not eliminate or come in conflict with the exterior reality; it remains for him exactly that which it must be: "an exterior world in brackets." (IV, 306)

Very much in the manner of phenomenology's anti-empirical position, Van Ostaijen finds exterior reality inconsequential unless one comprehends the presence of a much profounder world behind the exterior façade of objects. Like Husserl, Van Ostaijen does not dispense with the intellect, but considers it an aid for the exteriorization of reality in order to disclose reality's "aspect mystérieux." Van Ostaijen seems to be describing here a parallel formulation of Husserl's *Wesenschau*. One hardly needs to point out the astonishing similarity between Van Ostaijen's concept of exteriorization and Husserl's *Einklammerung* in the following quotation.

Situer l'extérieur dans la conscience de l'extériorisation, c'est spiritualiser cet extérieur empirique, la matière. Aussitôt qu'on aura vu selon cette vision, ne fût-ce qu'une seule fois, on ne cherchera pas d'autres merveilles que la réalité même: le merveilleux objet qu'est le moi enfermant en soi une table, une bouteille. Au lieu de niveler la vision et la pensée et bien loin d'exclure le merveilleux, la connaissance nous le révèle. Il n'est plus nécessaire d'être mage ou spirite. L'aspect fantasmatique des objets est une conséquence de l'état réel de notre connaissance. (IV, 137)

This and previous and subsequent correlations to important philosophical, artistic and aesthetic developments of the modern era remain intriguing enigmas in the study of Van Ostaijen. How much *did* he know of these developments when they were either beginning to blossom or were only in experimental stages? A clear answer remains wanting. The only provisional source one can point to for the philosophical basis of Van Ostaijen's poetics is his acquaintance with Salomon Friedlaender (Mynona). Perhaps this independent spirit, but devout Kantian, influenced Van Ostaijens' intellectual development more than can be ascertained at this time. One must remember, for example, that Husserl's philosophy owes a debt, as does much of modern German philosophy, to "Himmanuel" as Van Ostaijen called Kant with respectful disrespect.

Basically, Husserl's philosophy simply states that things are given, that they appear to our consciousness without us having to decide whether their autonomy is reality or appearance. A phenomenon is simply *there*. For Van Ostaijen the created organism of a work of art is also simply *there*, without any relations to anything exterior to its autonomous existence; it is "un organisme aussi réel qu'une fleur et qui, n'ayant pas d'équivalent dans la nature, n'est subordonné à aucune comparaison avec celle-ci." (IV, 143) The Polish philosopher Bochénski points out that for Husserl each individual object has a *Wesen*, an essence. Husserl's investigation is an "eidetic science which aims at the *intuition of essence*, the vision of the *eidos* (*Wesenschau*)." Van Ostaijen seems to speak essentially of a similar process in a discussion of modern painting.

Non seulement la surprise devant la réalité inconnue qui est un résultat intuitif de la connaissance consciente, mais aussi le mystère de cette réalité qui est la possibilité de la connaissance du monde extérieur, élimine les aspects multiples. Comme le mystère de la possibilité importe, il ne permet plus au sujet de dévier dans une aperception des éléments secondaires; cette connaissance de la possibilité fait se concentrer le sujet dans une aperception de la totalité. D'ailleurs: apercevoir dans un objet la possibilité de la connaissance subjective c'est le spiritualiser; or on ne saurait spiritualiser ce qui n'est qu'un détail, ce qui n'est qu'une qualité de l'objet, ou alors cette qualité, ce détail se concentre en lui-même, devient indépendant: une totalité. (IV, 141)

Van Ostaijen's inquiry here is akin to Husserl's intuition of general essences, phenomenology's transcendentalism. As Monroe Beardsley points out, such an investigation goes "beyond pure receptivity" and one "can recognize the particulars presented to him *as* particulars, and in so doing he can also grasp them as instances of universals." This is precisely what Van Ostaijen describes in terms of a *détail* (the particular) and a *totalité* (the universal).

Perhaps one could even argue for a parallelism in Van Ostaijen for Husserl's distinction between "sensual *hyle* (matter) and intended *morphe* (form)." Bochénski gives the following example. "In considering a tree, for example, one must distinguish between the meaning (*Sinn*) of the perception of the tree (its noëma) from the meaning of this perception as such (noësis) . . ." Van Ostaijen seems to make a similar differentiation for the act of creation; the distinction between the phenomenon as such and its transformation into art through an act of intuition which, as may be remembered, is also essential to Husserl's philosophy. Van Ostaijen is arguing against an empirical (what he calls "sensualistic") basis for poetry; that a poet 1) observes all the properties of a tree and 2) depicts the tree on the basis of this observation. But, Van Ostaijen insists, something is missing in such a process. What is lacking is a "lyrical-intuitive transposition of cognitive-theoretical knowledge; that besides the experience of the phenomenon tree, I also experience my perception of this tree as a phenomenon." (IV, 119) He provides another example from a poem in his volume *The Signal* (*Het Sienjaal*, 1918); he refers to the line where he writes Marcel Schwob is "the voice of the Baptist" ("gij zijt de stem van de Doper"). "If someone would ask me the question: But how can a person be a voice, unless explained as a metaphor, I answer, the voice is my mode of experiencing the phenomenon Schwob, just as I articulate my experience when I say, this house is high." (IV, 131)

Husserl's central concept of his phenomenological investigation, *Wesenschau* or the "intuition of essence," appears also to be the basis for the poetics of the Flemish author. For Van Ostaijen a poem is not important because of its "intellectual structure, but through a relationship which can only be comprehended by intuition as the greatest truth." (IV, 271) To write poetry is the "articulation of the intuitive knowledge of the world." (IV, 292) Finally, when Van Ostaijen argues for a mystical foundation in his poetry, this does not necessarily mean a negation of Husserl's phenomenology. Thévenaz spoke of phenomenology's "ascesis of the mind," its "transcendentalism." The point seems to be that phenomenology's ascesis never transcends the reality of this world, though this does not need to exclude idealism. Bochénski says quite clearly that phenomenology's "object is essence (*Wesen*); that is, the ideal intelligible content of phenomena, which is seized immediately in an act of vision – in the intuition of essence (*Wesenschau*)." Hence Van Ostaijen's "mysticism" is in a sense an *Einklammerung* of traditional theological connotations. Freed from transphenomenal elements, it is a mysticism of things in our world of reality.

Peut-on créer volontairement une école mystique? Non certes, mais on peut, sans se proposer cette fin et cependant sans mystification, assez loyalement si j'ose dire, se servir de ses moyens d'extériorisation. Il ne faut pas oublier que dans notre intention un mysticisme dans les phénomènes remplace le mysticisme en Dieu et que, d'autre part, ce dernier s'exprime, chez les auteurs mystiques, surtout par un mysticisme réaliste, haussant les phénomènes par lesquels il se manifeste, à une ambiance visionnaire. Il y a une rencontre dans la mysticité des phénomènes qui nous permet, sans employer ce divin, d'user des moyens d'application subjective dans les rapports des phénomènes et des mots comme seuls l'ont fait les mystiques.[17]

Van Ostaijen's "mysticité des phénomènes" is a poetic counterpart to Husserl's philosophical "eidetic science."

the present discussion. His poems could be called verbalizations of "the mysteriousness of the ordinary and [of] the quite ordinary mysteriousness." (IV, 44)

For the poet the "poverty" of his material is words. The basis of Van Ostaijen's poetics is the word in isolation, in full resonance by itself and in vibration with other words within the organism of the lyric. The previously mentioned instance of the aseity of words in the poem is a case in point, which he later, in a short piece on Guido Gezelle, calls "phenomenon-words." (IV, 375) The basic phenomenological desire to see the world as it is without any obstructing barriers inherited by man is Van Ostaijen's desire and poetic practice of seeing phenomena anew. "Poetry is eternal, but a poem comes out of momentary tension: the desire to see things *for the first time.*" (IV, 114) To recapture a primacy of vision results in a "democratization" of all objects. Within the work of art, nothing takes precedence over something else, that is to say "a tin box is no less plastic than a marble column." (IV, 89)

Merleau-Ponty: The Wonder of Perception

The French phenomenologist Maurice Merleau-Ponty firmly insists on man's inextricable relationship with the world. "Nous sommes toujours dans le plein, dans l'être, comme un visage, même au repos, même mort, est toujours condamné à exprimer quelque chose (il y à des morts étonnés, paisibles, discrets), et comme le silence est encore une modalité du monde sonore."[21] Merleau-Ponty's most insistent formulation is that "nous sommes de part en part rapport au monde." The phenomenological "reduction" (bracketing of the world by Husserl, of concrete man by Heidegger) is for Merleau-Ponty a wonder "devant le monde." "La réflexion ne se retire pas du monde vers l'unité de la conscience comme fondement du monde, elle prend recul pour voir jaillir les transcendances, elle distend les fils intentionnels qui nous relient au monde pour les fair paraître, elle seule est conscience du monde parce qu'elle le révèle comme étrange et paradoxal." (PP, viii) It is Merleau-Ponty who preserves both the essential ambiguity and paradoxicality of the world perceived and the wonder when one finally approaches the essence of phenomena. "All consciousness, all knowledge, all human undertaking are drawn on an ever present substratum: the world, a world that is always already-there, radically primary."[22] But the subject, we, remains "trop étroitement prise dans le monde pour se connaître comme telle au moment où elle s'y jette . . ."; ". . . l'homme est au monde, c'est dans le monde qu'il se connaît." (PP, ix + v) Van

Ostaijen agrees: "Le sujet est dans les objets comme l'objet dans le sujet . . ." (IV, 136)

Consciousness, "prendre recul pour voir jaillir les transcendances" makes it possible for Van Ostaijen to admit that "il n'est plus nécessaire d'être mage ou spirite. L'aspect fantasmatique des objets est une consequence de l'état réel de notre connaissance." (IV, 137) Van Ostaijen makes an analogy with the German Primitives in painting, whose art could be called a realistic mysticism. "Pour les peintres bavarois il n'y a rien que ne soit mystérieux. Mais aussi: tout ce qui se manifeste est réel." However, they ignore "le doute" (IV, 140). For Merleau-Ponty, as well as for the later work of Van Ostaijen, ambiguity is an essential aspect of the world and our perception of it. Merleau-Ponty makes it quite clear that "l'expérience du corps propre . . . nous révèle un mode d'existence ambigu."; and ". . . je ne me connais que dans mon inhérence au temps et au monde, c'est-à-dire dans l'ambiguité." (PP, 231 + 397) For Merleau-Ponty, a phenomenological investigation of reality reveals an essentially ambiguous existence. Meaning is ambiguous for Merleau-Ponty, "mixed up with non-meaning." "But we take up this meaning, which is unreflected rationality, by reflexion; we prolong it, and each of our acts, each of our thoughts expresses or gives a meaning to the world, without ever expressing it completely." [23] Hence phenomenological investigations of being are never complete, are ever repetitive, are a never-ending circle. "L'inachèvement de la phénoménologie et son allure inchoative ne sont pas le signe d'un échec, ils étaient inévitables parce que la phénoménologie a pour tâche de révéler le mystère du monde et le mystère de la raison." (PP, xvi) This phenomenological inchoateness might explain the incipient nature of these prose pieces by Van Ostaijen. Almost all end on a suggestion of continuity (for example, "Lines"), an observation equally applicable to the later poetry of Van Ostaijen (for example, "Geology").

Phenomenology, the philosophical venture of "le retour aux phénomènes," is for Merleau-Ponty a philosophy of perception, attempting "to show that perception is our original relation to the world, 'a type of originary experience.'" [24] "Il ne faut donc pas se demander si nous percevons vraiment un monde, il faut dire au contraire: le monde est cela que nous percevons." (PP, xi) The perception of ontological phenomena makes "le monde [de la perception] comme berceau des significations, sens de tous les sens, et sol de toutes les pensées, le moyen de dépasser l'alternative du réalisme et de l'idéalisme, du hasard et de la raison absolue, du non-sens et du sens." (PP, 492) It is but a short step from such profundity of phenomenological perception to a mystical reverence for phenomena, a phenomenological mysticism not a religious one, already indicated in Husserl's doctrine of *Wesenschau*. Van Ostaijen relates this transcendental devotion to the world of phenomena to the poetic process.

Ecstasy: my word enters the phantasmatical of objects and penetrates into that essence, the furrows of which lie too deep for mere understanding. And precisely this ecstasy in the possibility of articulation, precisely this alone allows me to express the other ecstasy in the phantasmatical nature of the intuitive knowledge of the object. The process of the word saves the development of the phantasmatical of the object. And because the phantasmatical aspect of the intellect soon becomes the phantasmatical aspect of the word, I enter, rationally, into a surreality. A healthy situation is it not? one which may please those critics who inspect a poem the way a doctor inspects a patient. (IV, 320)

Van Ostaijen clearly relates the wonder of such a phenomenologist as Merleau-Ponty confronted by the world ("berceau des significations") to the poet's wonder at the lyrical process. Van Ostaijen: "Émerveillement: je m'étonne de mon pouvoir de suivre par mon utilisation du mot les phénomènes dans leurs valeurs les plus imperceptibles a la seule intelligence. Par l'émerveillement devant le mot je sauve au cours de son éxteriorisation mon émerveillement devant le phénomène. Devant la nécessité de l'extériorisation, je revis dans le processus du verbe les aspects actifs du phénomène."[25]

In view of such energetic enthusiasm, it comes as a surprise to find an undertow of discontent in Van Ostaijen's later poetry and prose. Van Ostaijen's devotion to the reality of this world was genuine. Yet here lies exactly the crux of the problem. Van Ostaijen's awe of the innocent, virginal simplicity of the infinite riches of the world's phenomena forced upon him the sad realization that language is incommensurable with reality. The negative capability of language was both an incentive to create and a cause for discontented resignation. Van Ostaijen wanted to create a verbal object (the poem) as complete as a natural phenomenon. He knew he could not achieve this, yet neither would he relinquish the striving to fulfill this impossible dream. So keenly aware of the positive beauty of reality, he also sensed a foundation of nothingness. Heidegger accentuates the poet's capacity for expressing the negative aspect of existence, which places him (from Heidegger's point of view) on the same exalted level as the philosopher, because both are capable of perceiving and expressing nothingness, something which remains a "horror and an absurdity for science."

Just as the grotesques are an expression of Van Ostaijen's sense of incommensurability between this society and an order which should be, so are the posthumous lyrics and these prose pieces creations of an attempt at perfection which knew its failure in the act of creating. "A poem is never

as perfect as is a mammal with a finally severed umbilical cord." (IV, 316)
On the one hand, "the knowledge of the world is ... not accepted as an
existing unity, but the poet does strive gradually to penetrate it," (IV, 292)
and on the other, the fact that "for me, no single poem about the phenomenon 'fish' could ever be more powerful than this word *fish* itself."
(IV, 316) Throughout these prose pieces, and concurrently in the final
lyrics, there is always this dichotomy between reality and reflection
(language), between perfection and incompleteness, between ecstasy and
disillusionment. From this state of never resolved tension poetry is born.
"From a nostalgia for a native land of perfect knowing and from the realization of the vanity of every human attempt to reach it, from this double
cause of longing and powerlessness ... sprouts poetry." (IV, 316–7)
Merleau-Ponty touches obliquely on the discrepancy between the immu-
table fullness and independence of the object and one's perception of it.
Perception ". . . m'ouvre à un monde, elle ne peut le fair qu'en me dépassant et en se dépassant, il faut que la 'synthèse' perceptive soit inachevée,
elle ne peut m'offrir un 'réel' qu'en s'exposant au risque de l'erreur, il est
de toute nécessité que la chose, si elle doit être une chose, ait pour moi des
côtés cachés, et c'est pour quoi la distinction de l'apparence et de la réalité
a d'emblée sa place dans la 'synthèse' perceptive." (PP, 432)

Bachelard: Towards a Phenomenology of the Imagination

The essays on the philosophy of poetry by Gaston Bachelard combine phenomenology with metonymic art and correlate in various aspects to Van
Ostaijen's theory. Bachelard's essays on the four archetypal elements and
space constitute a formulation of an ontology of the imagination. Bachelard's discussion of the poetic imagination has a phenomenological basis in
that the poet seeks, at the same time, both the intimacy of phenomena and
of images. "Il veut exprimer l'intimité d'un être du monde extérieur."[26]
Akin to Merleau-Ponty's notion of ambivalence is Bachelard's insistence
on the imagination's ambivalent synthesis which unites dialectically "le
contre et le *dans*" of images. Images, as well as the work of art, are autonomous, a connection reiterated by Van Ostaijen throughout his essays. For
example: 'The work of art is an organism. *The work of art is a living
entity*. As such it is individual *an-sich* in the primary meaning of the word,
an-sich inseparable." (IV, 84) Bachelard's "matière imaginée" corresponds
to Van Ostaijen's "matière sensibilisée." Reminiscent of Bachelard's theory
of oneiric language is Van Ostaijen's statement that ". . . la poésie comme
tout autre art, est de la matière sensibilisée. Et sa matière est le mot avec

toutes les possibilités de son affectation au subconscient." [27] Just as phenomenology places the phenomenon before the act of thought, Bachelard's
"phénoménologie de l'image" places "l'image *avant* la pensée." [28]

In his final works Bachelard found it necessary to attempt a description
of the poetic imagination not merely through objective references to archetypal elements, but to "éclairer philosophiquement le problème de l'image
poètique, à une phénoménologie de l'imagination." [29] In a sense, this attempt is an extension of Merleau-Ponty's and Heidegger's preoccupation
with language, but now firmly embedded in the poetic imagination alone.
Bachelard's image, whose existence "est toute dans sa fulgurance, dans ce
fait qu'une image est un dépassement de toutes les données de la sensibi-
lité," [30] recalls Van Ostaijen's concept of aseity. *"The marvel of the primordial act of seeing urges aseity:* the drawing of a fish, the possibility of
expressing the phantasmatic, is felt as a maximum which cannot be dreamt.
*The elementary quality of aseity is specified by the wish to preserve the
phantasmatic.* In such a manner, the saying of words like *fish, tree, water,
air* is a maximum for the poet; the most positive of dreams." (IV, 242)

Central to Bachelard's phenomenology of the imagination is his concept
of the image. We must be able to grasp its specific reality. "L'image, dans
sa simplicité, n'a pas besoin d'un savoir. Elle est le bien d'une conscience
naive. En son expression, elle est jeune langage. Le poète, en la nouveauté
de ses images, est toujours origine de langage." [31] For Van Ostaijen it is
"through the communication of unknown resonances that the poet is new
and that he shows us things as if they were freshly minted." (IV, 319)
Curiously enough, Bachelard shows a disdain for metaphoric language
similar to Van Ostaijen. The metaphor, says Bachelard, is "un *image
fabriquée* ... une expression éphémère ou qui devrait être éphémère, em-
ployée une fois en passant ... ," while the image is an "... oeuvre pure de
l'imagination absolue, est un phénomène d'être, un des phénomènes speci-
fiques de l'être parlant." [32] As we saw before, Van Ostaijen is quite as
adamant in his denunciation of the metaphor.

I call the metaphor an intruder with the manners of a non-commissioned
officer. Its appeal to intelligence is an unpleasant dissonance in lyricism and that
sort of method of "you left, the others right" of the comparing and the compared
term disturbs my closed lyrical emotion ... I want equality by right and in fact
for all parts, and not a situation in which I try to make one oaf plausible by
giving it another to take along as a companion. (IV, 322–3)

May one see proof, in this parallel denunciation of metaphoric language,
that Jakobson's thesis of metonymic art as the basis for modern art has
something of the visionary about it? For, again, the following description
of the poetic process by Bachelard, which corresponds closely to Van

Ostaijen's, includes the implicit formulation of contiguity. Bachelard finds a dynamism in the lyric which, starting with an initial image, pulsates forward by "véritables lois d'images successives, un véritable sens vital. Les images mises en série par *l'invitation au voyage* prendront dans leur ordre bien choisi une vivacité spéciale qui nous permettra de désigner ... un *mouvement de l'imagination*." [33] What Bachelard calls "l'image initiale" corresponds to Van Ostaijen's "la phrase prémisse," and Bachelard's "mouvement de l'imagination" to Van Ostaijen's "lyrisme à thème." Van Ostaijen's outline of his poetic theory in "Un debat littéraire" closely resembles Bachelard's theory. "Je tends vers ce lyrisme que j'appele *pur,* qui, ayant posé une phrase prémisse et rien que cela, se développe d'une facon dynamique par les répercussions des mots dans le subconscient; celui-ci livrera à la conscience la matière nécessaire à la continuation et a l'achèvement de l'édifice, tandîs qu'en retour il sera du devoir de la conscience, de veiller à ce que cette matière reste dans les limites posées par la phrase prémisse." [34]

Finally, two central ideas of Bachelard's theory coincide with the poetic process of these prose pieces. Though empiricists in literary study might dispute its relevance, Bachelard emphasizes the unconscious aspect of creation, the dreaming into "la matière imaginée." His theory of poetry as oneiric language, a problem for methodological classifications, applies very well to Van Ostaijen's lyricism in these prose pieces. The poet seems to be dreaming himself into the heart of the subject matter, and awakens to a realization of profundity which hints at a nightmarish venture. In the domain of the imagination, according to Bachelard, images are proud masters bestowed with a divine right of kings. "Alors s'impose le réalisme de l'irréalité. On comprend les figures par leur transfiguration. La parole est une prophetie. L'imagination est bien ainsi un au-delà psychologique. Elle prend l'allure d'un psychisme précurseur qui *projette son être*." [35] The poet's dream has the quality of a daydream, as in most of these prose pieces by Van Ostaijen. 'Le poète vit une rêverie qui veille et surtout sa rêverie reste dans le monde, devant les objets du monde. Elle amasse de l'univers autour d'un objet, dans un objet." [36] The art of Van Ostaijen, his lyrics as well as these prose pieces, would have provided Bachelard with ample documentation for his phenomenology of the imagination.

FRANZ KAFKA AND PAUL VAN OSTAIJEN

Phenomenology has been a speculative basis for Kafka studies for some years now. Wilhelm Emrich, in his study of *Franz Kafka* (1958), goes so far as to state that Kafka's interpretation of being "erinnert... bis ins Detail an die moderne Fundamentalontologie Martin Heideggers und legt es nahe, Kafka als Vorläufer dieser Philosophie zu sehen und sein Werk im Anschluss an Heidegger zu interpretieren." A recent study links Husserl's phenomenology with Kafka's art. "A close comparison between the assumptions about the way man can know his world evident in *Der Prozess* and the basic assertions of Husserl will show... some striking similarities." [31] Comparative studies of Kafka's work and existentialism, the modern preoccupation with the absurd, and many other varieties of modern thought have already been made. Surely one could defend a thesis of Kafka's writings as metonymic art, in Jakobson's sense of the term. Kafka's work remains 'open' enough to allow future generations to annex the Kafkaesque hero to as yet undiscovered interpretative possibilities.

Clearly this is not the place to embark upon a lengthy speculation about a possible influence of Kafka on Van Ostaijen's prose writings. The eminent Belgian Kafka scholar, Herman Uyttersprot, has already noted some possible correlations. [38] Hidden in a footnote of the most recent full-length study of Van Ostaijen's poetry lies the contention that Van Ostaijen's translations of five early prose pieces by Kafka brought about a "new *unheimlich* genre of analysis," which should be particularly evident in the *Four Prose Pieces* and "Obsequies." [39] Such speculations, either fruitful or fruitless, have as yet not been subjected to a methodical investigation. Judging from the overwhelming critical literature on the German Proteus of modern literature, one may safely conclude that a comparative study of Kafka and Van Ostaijen would be just as feasible as other efforts of a far more speculative nature. A discussion of Van Ostaijen's prose work can never ignore the presence of Kafka, simply because of Van Ostaijen's translations of five pieces from *Betrachtung* (1913) to mark the German writer's death in 1924, which inspires a retrospective speculation about Van Ostaijen's acquaintance with Kafka's published work. Despite this fact, the following remarks are primarily from the point of view of Van Ostaijen's work and for the benefit of inclusiveness.

Van Ostaijen's Translations of Kafka

The Kafka translations by Van Ostaijen are naturally the most interesting fact in this discussion. Translated in 1924 and published in May/June 1925 as an act of commemoration, these pieces make Van Ostaijen eligible for the claim to be among the very first translators of Kafka in a foreign language. Certainly such a claim should be of interest to Kafka students

and a cause for pride in the critical sagacity of Paul van Ostaijen for those
who study his work. As far as can be ascertained, the Czech translations
by Milena Jesenská were first, followed by Van Ostaijen and a Spanish
translation of "The Metamorphosis" as close seconds.[40] It is but another
instance of Van Ostaijen's astounding familiarity with the most advanced
literary and artistic developments of his time.

The five "poëmata" wich, Van Ostaijen hopes, will show Kafka's "su-
perior spiritual attitude" are, in the order in which he presented them,
"Zum Nachdenken für Herrenreiter," "Wunsch, Indianer zu werden," "Die
Vorüberlaufenden," "Zerstreutes Hinausschauen," and "Der plötzliche
Spaziergang." The translations are literal and exact, with no significant
changes which might indicate an interpretative preference on the part of
Van Ostaijen. There is no record of why Van Ostaijen chose particularly
these pieces, considered juvenilia by critics, and not the maturer and more
essential texts, such as those collected in 1919 under the title *Ein Land-
arzt,* for example. The eighteen pieces of *Betrachtung* are, critically considered, not among the best examples of Kafka's art. Politzer calls them
"sketches," "five-finger exercises," which begin at "random and indicate
their end, if at all, only by a slight rise in emphasis ... Although "Meditation" abounds in colors (pastel) and figures (vague) and gives an early
example of Kafka's skill in packing a multitude of sensations into one
evenly sustained sentence, it is far from 'divine,' the term with which Brod
hailed the book. Rather it is a hodgepodge of reminiscences and promises,
an odd assortment of paragraphs, gleaned from a poet's imaginary diary."[41]
An explanation for the problem of Van Ostaijen's selection must remain
tentative and conjectural. The most obvious possibility is simply personal
preference. Or one could doubt Van Ostaijen's alleged familiarity with
Kafka's maturer work. The latter will remain a question mark, while for
the former possibility there is some evidence.

Even if one does not agree with Hadermann's contention that these
translations had a definite influence on *Four Prose Pieces,* some similarities
between these works of the two authors will become apparent. Van
Ostaijen was particularly sensitive to subtle seasonal changes, as many
lyrics and these prose pieces will affirm. Kafka's "Zerstreutes Hinausschaun" shows a similar registration of the barely perceptible alterations in
the atmosphere and light of spring as does Van Ostaijen's "O Thou, My
Splendid Solitude." The precision with which Kafka describes the phenomenon of shadow under changing light reminds one of the acute notation in "Obsequies" and the psychical importance of shadow in "Nicolas." "Wunsch, Indianer zu werden" describes attaining what Van Ostaijen

always strove for, the perfection of purity, such as the act of "pure" throwing away of money in "Anais." The final impact of Kafka's piece, one single sustained sentence, is having achieved a) a boy's dream of being an Indian riding bareback across the prairie, b) the unity of horse and rider and c) the perfection of unhampered motion itself. "Die Vorüberlaufenden," with its familiar Kafkaesque theme of irrational fear, might be compared to the more profound existential fear of "Nicolas."

These five pieces also share Van Ostaijen's preoccupation with both a purity of joy as well as a sense of foreboding (*Unheimlichkeit*). "Zum Nachdenken für Herrenreiter," with its typical Kafkaesque theme of frustrated striving, "Die Vorüberlaufenden" and "Zerstreutes Hinausschaun" conquer this foreboding of potential danger with the victory of light over shadow in that, when the man and his shadow have passed, "das Gesicht des Kindes ist ganz hell." One might even venture to suggest a predilection by Van Ostaijen for "Die Vorüberlaufenden," which combines fear and frustration with a tenuous rationalization, a theme also to be found in the grotesque "The Kept Hotel Key," without the ironic apology, however, for the feeling of impotence in the last two sentences of Kafka's piece.

Finally, there might have been an appreciation of the poetic style of these "sketches" as Politzer calls them. Though perhaps without the force of Van Ostaijen's work, these five pieces appear to describe the attempt to formulate the essential core of moods and feelings. In terms of Kafka's total achievement they might perhaps be called slight exercises for future more complex and consummate orchestrations. But for Van Ostaijen they might have shown primarily a poetic manner "de penser les choses"; that is, share his own mode of vision. Significantly, Van Ostaijen calls these pieces "poëmata," which is an apt term for a piece of creative prose of strongly poetic character. *Poëma* designates neither a poem nor a work of prose; it is what the *poeta* (the *agens* of the Greek verb *poiein*) makes or constructs. In English this leads etymologically directly to "poem," but in Dutch there is a better translation. Van Ostaijen, an avid reader of *Van Dale* (the Dutch equivalent of the *OED*), found *poëma* in the Dutch dictionary translated by "dichtstuk" rather than "gedicht" (poem). Van Ostaijen's *poëmata,* as the prose pieces discussed in this chapter are henceforth called, will indicate that the choice of the Flemish translator seems to have been a personal one, which concurred with his own vision at the time when he paid tribute to the memory of Franz Kafka. One may never get closer to the problem of the selection when considered from the point of view of the Kafka expert. Viewed from the standpoint of the student of

Van Ostaijen, the question may merely resolve itself in the simplicity of personal preference.

Kafka's Irreverent Mythology as Opposed to Van Ostaijen's Living Myth of the Sirens *

A discussion of Kafka and Van Ostaijen in terms of possible influence should include two pieces which both treat a similar mythical theme in an unorthodox manner: Van Ostaijen's "The Sirens" ("De Sirenen") and Kafka's "Das Schweigen der Sirenen." Kafka's tale reads like one of his characteristic paradoxical parables. Indeed, it sets out to prove an ironic paradox: "Beweis dessen, dass auch unzulängliche ja kindische Mittel zur Rettung dienen konnten." Odysseus makes elaborate preparations to withstand the lure of the Sirens' song, only to be reduced to an absurdity by their silence. He becomes preposterous, straining not to hear the Sirens, not to give in to their luring voices. "Odysseus aber, um es so auszudrücken, hörte ihr Schweigen nicht, er glaubte, sie sängen, und nur er sei behütet, es zu hören." The ironic "Anhang," which purports to set everything right by insisting on Odysseus' legendary craftiness, does not eradicate the graphically absurd figure of the Greek hero, bound to the mast, with wax-locked ears, straining to withstand their vocal magic, only to sail past Sirens who are utterly silent.[42] Kafka's irreverence towards the Greek myth is typical of his attitude towards ancient mythology.

Van Ostaijen, however, does not set out to be caustically paradoxical, but weaves a carefully constructed *Dichtung* around the double meaning of the word itself, a structure similar to his "lyrisme à thème," with the word *siren* as "phrase prémisse" and its ambiguity of meaning skillfully developed by poetic association. He plays with *Siren,* the mythological monster part woman, part bird, who lured seamen to their death by singing, and *siren,* a modern acoustical instrument which produces a piercing sound. The siren in the latter sense is particularly associated with ships and harbors. It is by now a commonplace that ships' sirens have a mournful, wailing tone when they whistle the ship's departure.

The first difference between Van Ostaijen and Kafka is that Van Ostaijen does not refer back to the time of mythology. The Sirens were caught "not so long ago," "a few miles south of the Azores." (III, 244) The harbors where they are brought are sprawling modern complexes – Lisbon, Liverpool, Rotterdam. The group of sailors who caught them were

* A complete translation of the *poëma* discussed in this section can be found in the Appendix.

"literally deaf," a straightforward and practical solution to the ancient peril. The piece is firmly rooted in the present; the existence of the Sirens is a matter of course. Only one slight but telling change is made in the original Homeric myth. The Sirens caught by Van Ostaijen's sailors whistle, they do not sing. Without ever mentioning the modern instrument, Van Ostaijen subtly transforms the captured Sirens into sirens. Sailors are practical. This is the only cause given for their turning the captured Sirens into utilitarian commodities. "A round opening was made in the wall of the sirens' brig and from this opening a pipe carried the sirens' whistling far above the deck, above the sea, above the stream and the city." (III, 244) In order to regulate their whistling to please the seaman's schedule, they prick them with needles, at the end of a lance, dipped in poppy juice. For poppy juice "when absorbed, produces an indescribable longing for space and an unlimited sadness. In sirens it awakens their past of distant seas, their former power over men and an ultimate sadness in which, as in another dimension, lie all of space and all delusions of power." (III, 244) Under the influence of the poppy juice, the Sirens' piercing scream hangs "suspended above the stream and the city."

This iteration of harbor and stream firmly associates the Sirens' presence and power primarily with harbors and ships. Factories situated in the country have also bought some of the captive Sirens, but "no matter what they try, they are not able to bring the sirens to make the plaintive wailing, which these animals aboard ship let out." (III, 245) Two major themes emerge. Van Ostaijen maintains the Sirens' (and sirens') close association with the sea, without which they fall silent and pine away; he also uses them as symbols of his theme of never fulfilled longing expressed, for example, with particular relevance to this story, in the poem "Geology."

Van Ostaijen does not take the Sirens' power of allurement away. Those "who have once heard the whistling of the sirens high over the city, for the rest of their lives cannot suppress their longing for this lament. They have, like the mouse to the cat, fallen prey to the harbor, where they know the ships and the sirens." (III, 245) Even in captivity, the Sirens realize their Homeric threat that "No life on earth can be/Hid from our dreaming." The theme of the Sirens in Van Ostaijen is diametrically opposed to Kafka's treatment, in that Van Ostaijen preserves their power, does not use them for ironic treatment of an ancient myth and hero and finally admits his attraction to them as personal symbols of his primary poetic preoccupation, the longing for poetic perfection and the nostalgic failure to achieve it.

Notice that Van Ostaijen never makes a metaphoric comparison between

Siren and a ship's siren. They *are,* within the poetic organism, one and the same thing. Van Ostaijen, trying to capture in words the purely personal meaning of the ship's sirens in the harbor of Antwerp, dreamed himself back, via the symbolic resonance of a single word, to the ancient myth, which gave expression to precisely the same feeling he encountered in a modern harbor town. The modern instrument has undergone the metamorphosis, not the legendary myth. Conversely, the ancient mythological figure has become a paradoxical poetic reality. The lure of the Sirens seems to stand for a symbol of the creative process, and the sailor, as in so many of Van Ostaijen's poems, for the poet. The reality of these specific poetic phenomena is graphically expressed in the little poem "Suicide of a Sailor" ("Zelfmoord des zeemans"), where the "Loreley" has the same powerful (here fatal) attraction.

> The seaman
> he hears the voice of the Loreley
> he looks at his watch
> and jumps into the water.

KANDINSKY'S THEORY AND VAN OSTAIJEN'S POËMATA *

A close similarity between Kandinsky's theory and Van Ostaijen's *poëmata* should come as no surprise to someone familiar with the work of the Flemish poet. The use of color in his lyrics is of great importance, though no one has paid any particular attention to it as yet. A prose passage such as the one describing Promethea in "Ika Loch's Brothel" provides ample evidence of Van Ostaijen's expertise in describing chromatic modulation. His lifelong interest in and acute understanding of the pictorial arts is not merely a biographical fact, but is amply documented by a series of theoretical essays. "Expressionism in Flanders" for example, contains a description of Paul Joostens' painting "Russian Madonna," displaying Van Ostaijen's competence in discussing such technical problems as color harmonies, relations of form and color, composition, and the effect of a painting on the spectator. The discussion of colors in this particular passage, as well as the entire essay, is clearly based on Kandinsky's work, *Über das Geistige in der Kunst* (1912), which he often quotes verbatim, and to which he constantly alludes. It is strange that such *poëmata* as "Curious attack," "Aquarelle" and the last paragraph of "Little Forest," have hardly been discussed, when such an obvious aid to their understanding is readily available. Hence it is only logical that a tentative ex-

---

* For a translation of the *poëmata* see the Appendix.

plication of these *poëmata* should start with Kandinsky's theory of painting.

"Curious Attack" or the Description of a Battle
between Abstract Colors

"Curious Attack" (III, 219–221) is a description of a battle, to be sure, but not between various "flower beds," nor even between colors which dominate such horticultural spaces, as one critic has suggested.[43] Borgers labelled it more accurately as the "only abstract painting in words" in the Dutch language. One should start interpreting "Curious attack" on its most basic level as a description of an abstract painting from within. The narrative first person singular has entered the painting, and is recording a peculiar contest of strength like a reporter covering a skirmish between two hostile army units. The combatants are colors, and the field of battle is the painter's canvas. Even a casual reader should realize that these particular colors have specific characteristics, which come into conflict with each other. There is more to these colors than meets the eye.

Contemplating colors, according to Kandinsky, affects a person in two ways. First there is the eye's vicarious enjoyment, as if mesmerized by the sheer beauty of color. It is merely a transient phase, since "die physische Wirkung der Farbe [wird] vergessen, wenn das Auge abgewendet wird."[44] More important than this elementary relationship of eye to color is the psychic action of colors in their beholder. Kandinsky sees the psychic impact of colors as axiomatic for modern art. "So ist es klar, dass die Farbenharmonie nur auf dem Prinzip der zweckmässigen Berührung der menschlichen Seele ruhen muss. Diese Basis soll als Prinzip der inneren Notwendigkeit bezeichnet werden." (UGK, 49) Pursuing the manner of this psychic effect, Kandinsky points to the principle of association as a possible explanation, though he refrains from assigning it scientific validity. Nevertheless he cannot help speculating about the important aspect of colors arousing senses other than sight alone; "Z.B. die rote Farbe kann eine der Flamme ähnliche seelische Vibration verursachen, da das Rot die Farbe der Flamme ist." (UGK, 46) Though being cautious about the principle of synaesthesia, which is based after all on association, it nevertheless permeates his subsequent discourse on painting. At this point Jakobson's theory of metonymic art and Kandinsky's formulation meet on common ground. For Kandinsky, color harmony is not only the fundamental pleasure of sight, but a *Berührung* of man's psyche, either directly or via sensory associations. Metonymic art, according to Jakobson, is controlled by *Berührungsassoziation*. Though one might quibble at this point that Kandinsky's use of *Berührung* has, perhaps, more the sense of being the impact of color on man's psyche, an examination of the entire book would argue for a retrospective proximity, if not similarity, to Jakobson's meaning of "contiguity."

Van Ostaijen speaks of a similar principle when he conceives of a poem as being "one chain of associatively bound realities" and of a painting as "placer l'un à côté de l'autre des plans et des objets à échelles diverses, sans indiquer la transition, soit par la perspective, soit par l'atmosphere; des objets à échelles differents se coupent comme s'ils étaient sur le même plan." (IV, 142) Hence, even in these abstract *poëmata* about colors, we find a threefold correlation between Kandinsky's theory of art, Van Ostaijen's theory and practice of poetry and art, and Jakobson's formulation of the metonymic pole of creative discourse. Indeed, one could even perceive of Kandinsky's chromatics and a number of Van Ostaijen's *poëmata* as an application of phenomenological perception in the area of pictorial arts.

For Kandinsky pure color (*die Farbe*) cannot exist independently of a representation of something, be it an object, space, or surface, while form can do so, either realistically or abstractly. Kandinsky is able to reduce form to its most elemental property as "Abgrenzung einer Fläche von der anderen." *Fläche* would correspond to Van Ostaijen's "valeur" (value). But this external description of form must immediately invoke an inner quality; hence form is also "die Äusserung des inneren Inhaltes." Pure color *an sich,* a paradigmatic red for example, can only be thought. For a color *to be* it must be materialized, that is to say, taking red as example: ". . . so muss es 1. einen bestimmten Ton haben aus der unendlichen Reihe der verschiedenen Rot gewählt, also sozusagen subjektiv charakterisiert werden und 2. muss es auf der Fläche abgegrenzt werden, von anderen Farben abgegrenzt, die *unbedingt* da sind, die man in keinem Falle vermeiden kann und wodurch (durch Abgrenzung und Nachbarschaft) die subjektive Charakteristik sich verändert (eine objektive Hülse erhält) . . ." (UGK, 54)

With this reciprocal relation between form and color, Kandinsky has unwittingly stated a chromatic phenomenology. Merleau-Ponty, true to his central idea of being "mêlés au monde," makes a similar statement in his phenomenological discussion of color and form. "En réalité, on a différentes fonctions de la couleur où la prétendue matière disparait absolument, puisque la mise en forme est obtenue par un changement des propriétés sensibles elles-mêmes." (PP, 353) Kandinsky's reciprocity between color and form finds a phenomenological equivalent: ". . . dans l'ensemble du champ visuel, par une sorte d'action réciproque ou chaque partie bénéficie de la configuration des autres, un éclairage général se degage qui rend à chaque couleur locale sa valeur 'vraie'." (PP, 360) Color and object are inextricably inter-mingled, according to Merleau-Ponty, echoing Kandinsky almost literally: "Une couleur n'est jamais simplement couleur, mais couleur d'un certain object . . ." (PP, 361) In short, for Kandinsky and for phenomenology, color becomes really significant when it assumes a form with specific attributes, when it is not static in its purity, but in a process of becoming, of action – "die Gegenwirkung der Form und Farbe."

Van Ostaijen applies this theory of reciprocity between form and color quite faithfully in "Curious Attack." The subjective character of rose for Van Ostaijen is apparently that of peace, which is enclosed in the objective "Hülse" of a square. The square is the only clearly delineated geometrical form, perhaps suggesting thereby the color's attributive function of "ob-jective peace." Even madder-carmine red, that is to say, a tone of red wanting to *become* (assume form) instead of *be,* before it changes into carmine, has a suggested semblance of form. This color is "arching and oscillating on the perimeter fragment." *Perimeter* is the significant word here, in the sense of being the outer boundary of a curved geometric figure. In German *perimeter* is *Flächenumriss,* in which sense it would be more closely associated with Kandinsky's most elemental formulation of form as "die Abgrenzung einer Fläche von der anderen." (UGK, 54) In other words, when the madder is first observed, it is fluctuating between color and form, having already realized itself into a semblance of the most rudi-mentary designation of form, which, at the same time, points towards the subjective qualities of carmine, in that its shape suggests a curve that can easily be developed into the more angular forms carmine assumes.

The double sense contained in "perimeter fragment" is repeated through-out the *poëma* by referring constantly 1) to its curved form ("arching," "arch," "archlike") and 2) wanting to become motion; i.e., wanting to change into carmine ("oscillating" "swaying" "exertion to oscillate" "to press immensely"). Even when the observer makes a humorous suggestion of what this spot of madder-wanting-to become-carmine looks like, Van Ostaijen preserves this distinction. "He could be a very baroque dachshund whose paws disappear in the belly." The choice of a dog with a long, rather shapeless body characterizes the impression which the spot of mad-der gives, while "baroque" is equally fitting in the sense of being irregular-ly shaped, applicable both to the form of the madder-shape as well as the rather odd-looking kind of dog. The fact that the "paws disappear in the belly" humorously emphasizes madder's inability to move.

Befitting its quality of sharpness, carmine becomes a beak "probably where line and perimeter fragment meet," which maintains carmine's relationship to madder. Carmine as beak, by association, becomes "sharp-bill" and, at the height of its aggression, "completely mouth." Also the second potential of madder, motion, is preserved in carmine's being "in turn as much as left leg, right leg." The subjective character of madder, its energetic aggression, which attempts to be formed through a curved, arch-like line, is materialized in carmine's mouth; "The arch form is an open mouth."

The blue, which has, according to Kandinsky, little potential *Steigerung*, and serves as a barrier between carmine and the rose square, has no more form than a "compact clump." The weak tint opaline has a negative formu-lation of shape; it has a "spine" formed by its "more pronounced tones." Only mauve has no assigned form. It seems to have primarily a function of allegiance to rose. Mauve is a delicate purple, and rose a delicate crimson or magenta. Purple and magenta are analogous harmonies on a painter's color-harmony chart. Mauve, being a chromatic kin, appears to be almost an alter ego of rose; it remains alert, while rose dreams its peace, rouses it when danger threatens, and is the mediary, harmonically, between rose, the other colors, and the values. Van Ostaijens hints at this role of mauve in the following series, which assigns the rose square its place in the total harmony of "Curious Attack": "Separated from the madder red by blue, opaline, mauve and manifold tremors of values lies the rose square."

Colors must obtain a definite chromatic tonality, be characterized sub-jectively according to the artist and to the color's innate attributes, and they are constantly in a process of *becoming* in relation to adjacent color values. The "Curious Attack" is executed by various tones of red. In Kandinsky's spectrum, paradigmatic red is a warm color of great energy and immense potential power. Materialized, red has a large range of possible forms. Van Ostaijen's madder (*kraplak*) corresponds to Kandinsky's *Krapplack,* which is a cold red of concentric power; i.e., usually in stable form. However, it harbors, but does not realize, a potential aggressive tendency; madder ". . . lässt eine Ahnung, ein Erwarten eines neuen energischen Aufglühens wie etwas, was sich in sich zurückgezogen hat, was aber auf der Lauer liegt und die versteckte Fähigkeit in sich birgt oder hatte, einen wilden Sprung zu machen." (UGK, 85) To realize this potentiality, the cold red must be-come brighter, at which point it gains *Körperlichkeit.* Van Ostaijen chooses the right tint, carmine-red, since it is, according to Kandinsky, neither a warm red nor a cold one, but "im mittleren Zustande." Carmine (Van Ostaijen's *karmijn* and Kandinsky's *Zinnober*) impresses one with its "scharfes Gefühl," it "zieht an und reizt," has "eine in sich sichere Kraft, die nicht leicht zu übertonen ist, die sich aber durch Blau löschen lässt, wie glühendes Eisen durch Wasser. Dieses Rot verträgt überhaupt nichts Kaltes und verliert durch dasselbe an seinem Klang und Sinn." (UGK, 83) The main actors have been delineated.

At the beginning of "Curious Attack," madder is stable. The potential aggression cannot be realized unless madder becomes a tint which can actualize this potentiality. Until the actual attack commences, madder remains energetic potentiality, attempting to realize itself into motion. The madder tries to 'formulate' its "versteckte Fähigkeit... einen wilden Sprung zu machen." (UGK, 85) "Inarticulate" in its fury and "apparently unavailing and unrelated" to its frustrated attempts at becoming, madder turns into carmine-red. True to Kandinsky's theory, the carmine-red attacks the blue, which separates it from its objective, the rose square. Carmine, as Kandinsky pointed out, cannot bear blue, a cold color. The attack on the royal blue meets with no opposition. Blue has a great quality of "Widerstandslosigkeit." The opaline is terrified by carmine's approach. Opaline, being a mixture of milky white and light blue, has not enough chromatic resilience to withstand an attack and, out of fear, dissolves in "an indeterminateness like the milky way." Now, when the carmine is ready to absorb the mauve – a delicate purple, a mixture of purple and rose – rose sees the danger, combines with the mauve, a chromatic ally, and foils carmine's design by dissolving into "neighbouring values."

Values in the context of "Curious Attack" have a very important function. Values are 1) distinct sections of color tones in relative relationship to the chromatic tonality of adjacent sections, or 2) may be seen as the basic expression of form ("Abgrenzung einer Fläche von der anderen"). Form, according to Kandinsky, is also "die Äusserung des inneren Inhaltes." (UGK, 54) Hence values do have their specific attributes in conjunction with correlative expressions of form and color within the context of the total painting. Values have their specificity which they, so to speak, may defend, but they are also susceptible to change; i.e., they may absorb colors sympathetic to their constituency. In "Curious Attack," values are both permeable and permanent. The rose square never relates to distant values, but only to those which are nearest, "the closest waves." When it escapes the carmine's attack, it "makes the leap into *neighboring* [italics mine] values." These values are congenial to rose and mauve, but impermeable to the force of carmine. "The carmine red winds up in the midst of the values. But the values are indeed impervious undulation. Where they become a hard resistance-proof mass, resilience compensates the lost ability of undulating. Hardened values evade the attack of the carmine-red through a hard resilient leap – like a flea."

Seemingly vulnerable to the boldness and force of such a strong color as carmine, the values cannot engage in direct combat, not being primary hues of equal strength. However, their strength lies in resilience which, according to the principle of contradiction, can be as effective as brute force. In fact, they engage in guerilla tactics against carmine's frontal attack: a "game-defense" which infuriates carmine all the more, but which it cannot counter. "If they at least would defend themselves seriously. So nasty: while playing to escape the danger of being gobbled up." It is not in the nature of values to be able to oppose an isolated color.

Within the anthropomorphic world of this abstract painting, carmine could directly attack even such a disharmonious opponent as blue in isolation: hue against hue. But values are, as it were, intermodulations of colors, an interplay of combinations of the color spectrum. This interplay constitutes the pictorial composition. "Auf dieser Harmonie fussende Komposition ist eine Zusammenstellung farbiger und zeichnerischer Formen, die als solche selbstandig existieren, von der inneren Notwendigkeit herausgeholt werden und im dadurch entstandenen gemeinsamen Leben ein Ganzes bilden, welches Bild heisst." (UGK, 77) The harmony of the values withstands the brute force of the intruder; carmine, by virtue of the harmonious interplay of the compositorial values, has overreached itself and will be defeated. Carmine, used to conventional warfare, has no way to cope with the guerilla tactics of the values. Balance is maintained despite its efforts. Subtler forces have triumphed over brutish energy. Defeated, carmine-red, forced by the composition's reciprocal harmony, must return to a stabler red. "The carmine red is again madder."

In terms of Kandinsky's values of colors, blue should have been playing the role of rose in "Curious Attack." "Sehr tiefgehend entwickelt das Blau das Element der Ruhe." (UGK, 77) Rose is specifically Van Ostaijen's choice. The rose square is "at peace" and "lies island-secure in values." For Van Ostaijen, rose seems to have a quality of tenderness and peace as in his poem "Irrelevant Polka" ("Onbeduidende polka"). Yet it is also vulnerable, just like the "threadbare rose" of Colombine in the poem. In "Curious Attack" rose has a precarious dreamlike quality, totally dependent on the perilous security of the other colors. When carmine has shown itself to be a realistic threat, rose awakens, as it were; "dream befalls the miscalculation in the certainty of the unconditionally being separated." When its precarious peace is assaulted, rose is forced to awaken to its true attributes: its vulnerability and its strength. "To drive strength to center, a moment, to conquer desperation." The rose square was in a disharmonious relationship with its own values, while the carmine was so in relation to the total composition of this world of colors.

Even for this choice of rose one might find possible explanations in Kandinsky's theory. Blue is the color of peace, of metaphysical profundity. The tranquility of blue is spiritual and effects its force profoundly inwardly. Blue is not vulnerable in the way rose is in "Curious Attack." At its extreme poles it can either be "einer nicht menschlicher Trauer" (dark blue) or proceed "bis es zur schweigenden Ruhe übergeht" (light blue). "Das Blau wird schwer akut und kann nicht zu grosser Steigerung sich heben." (UGK, 78) Kandinsky's description of blue is analogous to Van Ostaijen's royal blue in "Curious Attack." The royal blue does not take any measures against carmine's attack; it does not undergo any *Steigerung*. It remains seemingly unaffected when "half of the carmine-red sticks right into the clump of the royal blue." Similarly, the blue tones in the opaline, which Van Ostaijen calls its "spine" or "more pronounced tones," weaken and dissolve. The blue, by its given psychic nature, cannot and will not defend itself. Rose does. Part of its realization, its awakening to its potentialities, is its "crimsonness"; rose being a mixture of magenta (a brilliant crimson) and white. Blue is concentric, red eccentric in movement. Movement is crucial to rose, in order to evade carmine's attack. This movement (*Steigerung*) lies at its center; is active in its crimson kernel. Blue's passivity would have prevented it from foiling the red assault because of its contemplative nature and its refusal to act. Blue *is*; it cannot *become*. Blue is a more veracious color for peace than rose, since it has the character of *Vertiefung,* as opposed to rose's *Träumerei.*

Since red dominates "Curious Attack," movement is prominent in this *poëma.* This abstract world of colors has a remarkable dramatic quality one would hardly expect from such irrational, anarrative material. As the title so aptly notes, a mysterious force evokes a presentiment of fear in the reader by its aggressive implications. Carmine's zeal to devour rose is hardly cause enough, in dramatic terms, to warrant such undeniably bellicose dynamism. There is no meaningful reason or goal behind this strife. Yet, even when viewed as simple motion, the *poëma* forces its attention upon us and appears meaningful. "Curious Attack" could be seen as simply a remarkable verbalization of motion. The circular movement of "Curious Attack" corresponds to what Van Ostaijen calls the dynamism of a canvas; "the blood circulation of the canvas, regulator of the organic mechanism." (IV, 87) A work of art is completely independent, and can only be judged by its own psychic and material laws; each work of art has its own dynamism. *Dynamis* (force) seems to correspond to Kandinsky's "innerliche

Notwendigkeit," and Van Ostaijen insists on a sharp distinction between *dynamis* (force) and its result *kinesis*. "The inner energy of each organism is dynamic; whether this organism apparently moves or stands has nothing to do with dynamism. By dynamism we do not mean the representation of kinetic phenomena (Futurism). A standing man is surely no less the result of inner energy than one in motion. Both are dynamic, the latter kinetic." (IV, 87) Hence the movement of carmine, its kinetic progression towards the rose square, is a result of madder's dynamism, just as rose's escape, the leap into adjacent values, is a kinetic result of its crimson properties. The dynamism of "Curious Attack" in terms of its colors is largely based on Kandinsky. The *Bewegung* or kinetic progression, the resultant of the phenomena's dynamo, is in terms of verbal composition a metonymic art, a *kinesis* of contiguity. "Curious Attack" (as well as the other *poëmata*) is what Jakobson calls "ein Reich zu selbständigem Leben erweckter Metonymien."

Van Ostaijen's *poëma* incorporates many of the features of metonymic art as outlined by Jakobson in his article on Pasternak. Madder is a general metonymy of the color red; conversely, carmine is a kinetic metonymy of madder. What was explained before in terms of Kandinsky's theory can now also be seen as metonymic formulations; royal blue a metonymic expression of impermeable passivity, the rose square of the illusion of peace, etc. Despite the abstract nature of the piece, synecdochic details, which Jakobson finds characteristic of metonymic style, are used by Van Ostaijen. Madder is associated with dynamic movement which, as yet, has not been materialized, has not *become* kinetic progression. Madder is "arching," "oscillating," "to displace weight from left to right." Since the carmine carries out the madder's potential aggression in the attack on the other colors, the synecdochic details are more aggressive and relevant to Kandinsky's description of carmine's "scharfen Gefühls." Carmine is "beak," "direct sharpbill," "mouth."

Several of Jakobson's types of *Berührungsassoziation* are employed in this *poëma*. Metonymic methods such as whole to part can be seen in madder's potential and carmine's realization of aggression and movement; these metonymic transformations are also functional in terms of the color's organic *Notwendigkeit*. "Actively-organic he is always completely that organ which is just then functional. The carmine red is in turn as much as left leg, right leg, mouth." Part to whole movement can be seen in the final sentences, after the carmine has been foiled. "The carmine red oscillates mightily. The mouth becomes right leg again. Oscillation. Left right left. Left leg. The carmine red is again madder." Jakobson's "von der Ursache zur Wirkung" can be seen in ". . . how he oscillated, and now the beak. Direct sharpbill in the compact clump of the royal blue." The reverse of this, from effect to cause, appears in the lines immediately following: "The hardness of the royal blue greatly heightens the anger of the carmine red and, its inevitable result, its attack's sharpness. This happens suddenly; one half of the carmine red sticks right into the clump of the royal blue."

Many other correlations between Jakobson's theory and Van Ostaijen's practice could be enumerated. For example, the obviously similar metonymic method of "die Äusserung des Gegenstandes nimmt auf sich seine Funktion" in: "Exertion to oscillate. Presses immensely towards the right and becomes croplike malevolent when he notices the ungainliness of his organism . . . Inarticulate fury sticks in his – the madder red – throat. The throat must be swollen. Only nothing indicates it. Where is the throat." And surely "Curious Attack" as a whole illustrates Jakobson's formula that "die Abstraktion wird zu selbständigen Handlungen befähigt, und diese Handlungen werden wiederum vergegenständlicht . . ." That is to say, abstract red becomes madder and then carmine; their attributes of motion and aggression are in turn *vergegenständlicht* in "oscillation," "left leg," "right leg," "bill," "beak," "mouth," etc.

Metonymic art distorts the normality which would be expected within verbal compositions. Jakobson mentions under this heading, for example, the metonymic urge to efface precise demarcations of objects. Van Ostaijen is similarly reluctant to define with precision, but rather lets the cumulative effect of images carry the burden of meaning. The result is a curious vacillation between indeterminateness and precision, which must combine into a total effect, and should not have a reciprocal action of definition. "The madder-carmine red. Not abstract: the madder. He is extremely concrete. Yet I would not be able to say in what manner he is concrete. Only, it seems to me: arching and oscillating on the perimeter-fragment. Movement is: to displace weight from left to right and to oscillate." This is also an instance of a "beliebige Kontiguität" becoming a "kausale Reihe." Using Jakobson's striking phrase, one could call "Curious Attack" a *poëma* about the "metonymischen Wahlverwandtschaft" of colors.

The dramatic and dynamic quality of "Curious Attack" is perhaps its most striking feature. Kandinsky made a shrewd observation concerning the dramatic quality of movement in general. A seemingly pointless motion can contain a great dramatic intensity and a fearful mysteriousness. As soon as the motion has been explained in practical or utilitarian terms, it loses its mysteriousness and dramatic potential. One should be able to maintain, according to Kandinsky, a suspension of disbelief regarding even the most common objects in order to uphold their intrinsic mystery. "Eine sehr einfache Bewegung, von welcher das Ziel unbekannt ist, wirkt schon an und für sich als eine bedeutende, geheimnisvolle, feierliche. Und das, solange man das äusserliche, praktische Ziel der Bewegung nicht kennt." (UGK, 106) One may speak of such a *Bewegung* in "Curious Attack" since, obviously, a "practical objective" can hardly be argued. Kandinsky's formulation is, naturally, an apology for abstract art where with only color and abstract forms, he must produce this "bedeutende, geheimnisvolle, feierliche" effect. A similar result is evoked by a reading of Van Ostaijen's "Curious Attack." "In der einfachen Bewegung, die äusserlich nicht motiviert ist, liegt ein unermesslicher Schatz voller Möglichkeiten." "Curious Attack" has no discernible external motivation and is full of exegetical possibilities. The application of Kandinsky's theory of colors only induces a wide variety of possible interpretations.

In terms of *Bewegung,* the *poëma* is circular. The last line ("The carmine red is again madder") instantly invokes the first ("Stable he is madder"), and in no way prevents a recurrence of carmine's attack. Like a painting, it does not exhaust possibilities, but multiplies them. As phenomenology aims to do, the *poëma* does not want to "explain" objects, but rather understand their specificity while preserving their authenticity. The aura of creative mystery of the most common objects or phenomena which Kandinsky wants to preserve, is precisely what Van Ostaijen achieved in his final poems. "Sobald man sich aber erinnert, dass in unseren Strassen nichts Rätselhaftes vorkommen darf, so fällt im selben Augenblicke das Interesse für die Bewegung aus: der praktische Sinn der Bewegung löscht den abstrakten Sinn derselben aus." (UGK, 106) Van Ostaijen formulates this statement by Kandinsky, which essentially describes the poetic process, more succinctly as "the mysteriousness of the ordinary and the quite ordinary mysteriousness." (IV, 44) In quality as well as technique, these *poëmata* belong with Van Ostaijen's finest lyrics, capturing what Bachelard formulates as expressing "l'intimité d'un être du monde extérieur." The psychic attributes of colors have not been exhausted in "Curious Attack." The *poëma* gives a precedent of experiencing colors verbally in a new way, of experiencing colors on their own terms, as phenomena.

To provide a textbook definition of the meaning of "Curious Attack" is an impossible and fruitless task. In this discussion only certain correlative assumption were made to see the *poëma* as a phenomenological description of colors, based on Kandinsky's theory of painting. But in terms of its precise meaning it remains open, or subject to as many varied reactions as people have to a work of art. When it is no longer open in its potentiality of meaning, but closed through a uniform agreement on its meaning, the work of art *is* no longer *an sich,* but has become a fixed metaphor, its creative lifespan has been terminated, it has been reduced to a cliché. Kandinsky consequently champions a "Versteckte Konstruktion... nicht eine klar daliegende, oft in die Augen springende ('geometrische') Konstruktion, die an Möglichkeiten reichste bzw. die ausdruckvollste zu sein, die aus dem Bilde unbemerkt herauskommt und also weniger für das Auge als für die Seele bestimmt ist." (UGK, 112–3)

Kandinsky's "versteckte Konstruktion," realized verbally in Van Ostaijen's *poëma,* corresponds to metonymic art. For Kandinsky "diese versteckte Konstruktion kann aus scheinbar zufällig auf die Leinwand geworfenen Formen bestehen die wieder scheinbar in keinem Zusammenhang zueinander stehen: die äussere Abwesenheit dieses Zusammenhanges ist hier seine innere Anwesenheit. Das äusserliche Gelockerte ist hier das innerlich Zusammengeschmolzene." (UGK, 13) Jakobson formulates a similar principle in terms of poetics: "eine beliebige Kontiguität kann als kausale Reihe aufgefasst werden"; "die geschaffene Verbindung überschattet das zu Verbindende, beherrscht es"; "der Dichter definiert die Kunst als gegenseitige Ersetzbarkeit der Bilder." Again Van Ostaijen, Jakobson and Kandinsky are in agreement. One may even suggest a common denominator for them: Cubism as metonymic art. Jakobson singles out Cubism as being an exemplary metonymic art from, while Van Ostaijen, a lifelong champion of Cubism, calls Kandinsky the "lyrical pole" of the Cubistic style in painting. "Curious Attack" may thus be seen as a rare transferral of pictorial metonymy to verbal metonymy, without harming the characteristics of either medium. In short, "Curious Attack" is a Cubistic painting in words.

"Aquarelle": The Fingers' Dream and Their Abortive Rebellion

There are two other *poëmata* in which color plays an important, but not quite such an exclusive, role as in "Curious Attack." In both instances the influence of Kandinsky's theory of colors is clearly ascertainable. "Aquarelle" (III, 215) is the first of the *Four Short Tales* which also includes "Curious Attack." Starting out to paint verbally an abstract water-color, "Aquarelle" proceeds to describe the rivalry between tactual and visual senses. The psychic properties of colors in this *poëma* can again be traced to Kandinsky's treatise. Blue, for example, has in "Aquarelle" more clearly Kandinsky's characteristic of profound peace than it did in "Curious

Attack." Paradigmatic blue has a very strong "Vertiefungsgabe," and its physical (visual) movement is concentric. Van Ostaijen describes a similar value: "Blue rests... and determines the ratio inwardly-kernel." For Kandinsky blue, the cold, spiritual, concentric color, has the warm yellow as polar opposite, a color which visually moves eccentrically. An earthy color, yellow has a boisterous spontaneity and energy which tends towards "das Springen über die Grenze, das Zerstreuen der Kraft in die Umgebung" (UGK, 75–6) which can arouse, excite or even irritate a person. In Van Ostaijen's abstract watercolor, yellow "runs childlike desire for the solution of stability." Blue and yellow are Kandinsky's first set of chromatic opposites.

Red is present in "Aquarelle" in its abstract form, without the actualized tonalities such as madder or carmine, as in "Curious Attack." Kandinsky opposes red, in its paradigmatic state, to yellow in terms of their respective energies. Red "wirkt innerlich als eine sehr lebendige, lebhaftige, unruhige Farbe," but without yellow's frivolity in the spending of its energy. Though a color of movement (while blue is a color of rest), red concentrates its energy inwardly. Van Ostaijen mixes blue's *Vertiefung* and red's *Bewegung in sich* to obtain mauve, which combines concentric movement and a desire for spirituality, so that it can "vibrate far up to the limit of experience." The fingers have been attempting to experience tactually these psychic attributes of colors, a task which properly belongs to the eyes; i.e., qualities transformed via the act of vision into colors' "innerlicher Charakter als seelische Wirkung." (UGK, 72)

In the first paragraph the fingers have been stroking the paper, have been actually experiencing the colors purely in terms of fluidity. "Aquarelle floats red." "Around color bubbles swirls water." "Wattmanpaper flows mauve-saturated. The mauve water becomes grains of Wattmanpaper." But this is not enough for the fingers. They want "to go further to the knowledge of my eyes." They want to *feel* the colors' essential values: "to feel the peace of blue and to penetrate to the limit of ... mauve vibration." Following Jakobson's *Berührungsassoziation,* the fingers contiguously want to become eyes via the intermediary stage of taste, expressed metonymically as 'their wish is to be lips ... thirst at the well of orange." Again Van Ostaijen's choice of color is apt. Orange ("das warme Rot, durch verwandtes Gelb erhöht") transforms red's inward motion into "der Bewegung des Ausstrahlens, des Zerfliessens in die Umgebung," but due to red's dominance over yellow, orange retains "den Beiklang des Ernstes." (UGK, 85–6)

If one assumes Van Ostaijen's mauve to be like Kandinsky's violet (in

German mauve is translated as *hellviolett*), one finds that the colors of Van Ostaijen's "Aquarelle" correspond to Kandinsky's second set of contrasting basic, primitive color-tones. The diagram in Kandinsky's book starts with red ("Bewegung in sich") as central color, moving in one direction (enhanced by yellow) towards orange, and in the opposite one (enhanced by blue) towards violet. In the first two sentences of "Aquarelle" Van Ostaijen seems to follow this diagram quite closely. Red is mentioned first, central color in the diagram. Blue and yellow follow immediately afterward as a pair; in the diagram they are on either side of the red as polar movements: blue towards concentric, yellow towards eccentric movement. The first tint in the *poëma* is mauve (Kandinsky's violet), a mixture of red and blue. Kandinsky's violet "entsteht durch das Zurückziehen des Rot durch Blau . . . welches die Neigung hat, vom Menschen sich weg zu bewegen." "Violett ist also ein abgekühltes Rot im physischen und psychischen Sinne." (UGK, 86) Van Ostaijen's mauve also moves away "far up to the limit of experience." Mauve has an inner depth, which the fingers crave to sense. In the second paragraph orange is mentioned which, diagrammatically, has a greater component of yellow and is, therefore, "einem von seinen Kräften überzeugten Menschen ähnlich." (UGK, 86)

Van Ostaijen's choice of primary color tonalities in a basic opposition between two distinct sensory experiences seems to have been deliberate. The fingers are "naturally" more attracted to the more sensual yellow, orange, and even the red. All three colors share an increasing rate of eccentric movement, all three are warm colors. At the same time they are sequentially associated, according to Kandinsky, through the pivotal red with their polar opposites: blue and mauve (Kandinsky's *Violett*). The fingers crave a double intimacy; the more external, active values of yellow and orange, as well as the more passive, more profound intimacy of spiritual peace of the mauve and, ultimately, the blue.

In the second paragraph, the fingers have their brief reverie of the "striving to be eye." "This is the time of beauty for my fingers. Their total dissolution in their parasensual desire. They are no longer. They are only labile. They are becoming." For a moment the fingers are in that state of profound dreaming which Bachelard finds to be basic to the poetic process. In a sense, the fingers are dreaming themselves into *l'intimité des choses* (in this case the psychic values of colors) while they really can only touch. At this point the fingers are poets dreaming Bachelard's profound dream. "C'est en rêvant à cette intimité que l'on rêve au repos de l'être, à un repos enraciné, à un repos qui a une intensité et qui n'est pas seulement cette immobilité tout externe qui règne entre les choses inertes." [45] The ensuing demise of the fingers, when the eyes sense the fingers' rebellion, juxtaposes poetically Kandinsky's distinction between the physical and the psychical force of colors. As Van Ostaijen so aptly calls them, the fingers, dreaming of attaining the psychic intimacy of the colors, are "idealists of the transferral of the spiritual to the parasensual."

In the third paragraph "the eyes awaken" to the "uprising" of the fingers. Making their desire to be eyes "too real," the fingers were essentially dreaming. As usual, Van Ostaijen has a key term hidden, often abstract to preserve its incognito, which hints retrospectively at present development. *Labile* connotes being prone to lapse, to undergo change: instability. When the fingers were dreaming their dream of "striving to be eye," they were no longer fingers, and yet not quite eyes either. In this suspended state "they are no longer. They are only labile." But this is a precarious and vulnerable state, and the fingers are easy prey for eyes who "kill the things which dissolved themselves in the lability of too real desire." The eyes are dictators, and will not relinquish their specific function. Perception is a primary mode of comprehending phenomena. Goethe saw in his poems as well as in his theory of optics that "the eye and its acts are . . . the most decided representatives of a mode of understanding reality which is in a high degree creative." [46]

At the moment of defeat, a positive note is sounded by Van Ostaijen. The fingers profited from the experience of trying to become visual. Despite defeat, their dream had its purpose. This purpose was the trying, the striving to understand or experience the intimate attributes of phenomena. At least the fingers, though they "were always fingers," tried to realize their desire to pierce through into a realm superior to their own. They know that "they will never drink orange and never stroke mauve," but there is strength in their weakness. Like "Curious Attack" there is a circular movement of never ending striving. For the fingers' limitation does not prevent them from rebelling again; their limit is but a "temporary hypertrophy of their desire." This sense of perpetuity is underlined by the adverbial *perhaps* which combines possibility and uncertainty, and is used twice in succession in the fifth paragraph, which is only three sentences long. The last paragraph emphasizes again Van Ostaijen's sympathy through the conjunctive force of "yet despite weakness it is rebellion." There is positive resignation in the fact that "my fingers were able to vibrate for a moment . . . in the delusion of being labile and on the way to realizing their desire." The fingers dream an impossible dream, yet they cannot be forced by the dictatorial eyes to relinquish this dream, or prevent them from their futile attempt at realization. "Aquarelle" in that sense has the same feeling of ceaseless striving as "Curious Attack." There the implication is that the rose square will always dream its dream of objective peace, and that the madder will become carmine again to attempt to destroy it.

Another parallel can be found in "Anais" (III, 216–217), the second of the *Four Short Tales*. The model Anais knows that there is no such thing as "pure" throwing away of money. "The dissonance is clear between the psychic condition for this act – resignation – and the act itself – a positive rebellion with hope of salvation because of the rebellion." After she has performed the act of throwing away her monthly salary, there is "a dissatisfaction in her like a slight nightmare." Nevertheless, like the fingers in "Aquarelle," Anais "observed that discontent was the only possible form of contentment for her." The similarity between Anais' futile gesture, which could never equal a paradigmatic throwing away of money, and the fingers striving to be eyes, is all too obvious. The desire to penetrate into a paradigmatic realm and the knowledge of perpetual failure which, nevertheless, cannot kill the urge to try, is a theme basic to most of Van Ostaijen's later poetry, as it was in a slightly different guise in that one grotesque with a difference, "The Kept Hotel Key." Bachelard summarizes this theme as well as the plight and the pride of the fingers in "Aquarelle"; "Quand la main n'a pas la force, elle a la patience."

The Coda of "Small Forest": Colors of Equilibrium

The influence of Kandinsky's theory of colors can be traced in one more *poëma* of a later date. "Small Forest," (III, 249) which is the first of *Four Prose Pieces,* has a final paragraph of apparent complexity, where colors carry the burden of meaning. A coda, the paragraph reiterates the preceding movement from joy to despondency, but adds a final note of peace and tranquillity. The poet is lying on the forest's floor, letting his eye rove from the ground to the pines, back to the ground and a hay wagon, which suddenly has entered his field of vision. The entire psychic movement of the *poëma,* as well as the trajectory of the eye, is synthesized in one long final sentence after the introductory counsel: "You must lie on the ground." "Thus, across the ground, past much ochre and brown, past much green, your eye gains the bark and again the green, the old and the young and finally this grey, this crazy grey-green, which is so exhausting that your eye flees to earth and slowly, only slowly, awakens to the motion of a brown hay wagon in the midst of the yellow-brown bed of needles."

Brown is a *Vertiefung* of red through black, whereby the black reduces the inner glow of red to a minimum. As a color, brown has a barely perceptible movement towards the viewer, yet from this externally slight tonality "entspringt . . . ein lauter gewaltsamer innerer [Ton]." For Kandinsky brown has "eine unbeschreibliche inner Schönheit: das Hemmen." (UGK, 84) Ochre may be seen as simply a lighter shade of the warm browns. Green is an important color for Kandinsky and is, in his theory, the ideal mixture of yellow and blue. Green is the color *par excellence* of peace, an earthly (as opposed to blue's heavenly) self-satisfied peace. "Absolutes Grün ist die ruhigste Farbe, die es gibt: sie bewegt sich nach nirgend hin und hat keinen Beiklang der Freude, Trauer, Leidenschaft, sie verlangt nichts, ruft nirgend hin." (UGK, 78) Green has a beneficial effect "die auf ermüdete Menschen und Seelen wohltuend wirkt," and is the primary color of summer "wo die Natur die Sturm- und Drangperiode des Jahres, den Frühling überstanden hat und in eine selbstzufriedene Ruhe getaucht ist." (UGK, 79) The season of „Small Forest" is June.

After "his retina became threadbare from the maddest realities of light," the poet both visually and psychically returns to a state of tranquillity and peace. First through the brown which restrains the excesses of the spectrum and precipitates a *Vertiefung,* which becomes fully realized in the passive force of the mindless peace of green. By the "young" and the "old" green, Van Ostaijen is simply referring to the pines of June and the pines of winter. Now a note of dissatisfaction sets in with "finally this grey, this crazy grey-green, which is so exhausting." For the beneficial effect of green becomes tiresome after a while, its complete passivity strikes one as "einer Art Fettheit, Selbstzufriedenheit." (UGK, 79) To juxtapose green and grey is a natural consequence in terms of Kandinsky's theory. Both are characterized by immobility and restfulness. Grey's immobility is "trostlos." "Je dunkler dieses Grau wird, desto mehr Übergewicht bekommt das Trostlose, kommt das Erstickende zur Geltung." (UGK, 82) As an equilibrium of black and white, grey is a mechanical mixture. One can also obtain grey through an optical mixture of green and red. Exhausted by the double immobility and passivity of the grey-green, "the eye flees to earth." And when the eye awakens, as if from a drugged sleep, it awakens slowly "to the motion of a brown hay wagon in the midst of the yellow-brown bed of needles." Here the brown of the hay wagon arrests the excesses of grey-green's narcosis, just as before it checked the excess of light to allow green to soothe the retina. Between the two excesses of the "maddest realities of light" and the deadening impassive rest of the green, brown brings back a proper perspective, strikes a balance, with the aid of yellow, of a more joyous and profound nature. To the "unbeschreibliche innere Schönheit" of brown yellow adds an active, youthful and glad note. "Small Forest," like the other two *poëmata,* ends on a note of resigned acceptance of contented discontent.

In "Curious Attack," "Aquarelle" and the final paragraph of "Small Forest," Van Ostaijen gives poetic proof of having learned Kandinsky's lesson of an interdisciplinary action among the arts. In these *poëmata,* Van Ostaijen realized Kandinsky's vision of a movement in literature analogous to the one he was codifying for the arts. As color is to painting, so is the word to language; both are psychic values rather than physical ones. *"Das Wort ist ein innerer Klang.* Dieser innere Klang entspringt teilweise (vielleicht hauptsächlich) dem Gegenstand, welchem das Wort zu Namen dient. Wenn aber der Gegenstand nicht selbst gesehen wird, sondern nur sein Name gehört wird, so entsteht im Kopfe des Hörers die abstrakte Vorstellung, der dematerialisierte Gegenstand, welcher im 'Herzen' eine Vibration hervorruft."[47] This statement by Kandinsky is similar to Van Ostaijen's theory and practice, to phenomenological perception, and to Jakobson's metonymic art. Van Ostaijen called it a "lyrisme à thème" which transforms "la matière sensibilisée" into verbal art. From a phenomenological viewpoint Kandinsky is speaking of bracketing the object to obtain the transcendental essence of phenomena. Such a bracketing in poetic practice could be called a metonymy. As Jakobson clearly states, the metonymic principle in art and literature leads to a *Gegenstandslosigkeit.* The independently created *Verbindung,* a contiguity (Kandinsky's *Vibration*), becomes an autonomous *Gegenstand.* All three theories seem to share a common basis of a radically different mode of seeing and describing reality from what is commonly accepted as normal. Van Ostaijen's *poëmata* are the creative proof of the theoretical speculations.

PHENOMENOLOGICAL POËMATA
"Lines," "Nicolas," "Obsequies": The Realization of "Méontologie"

"Lines": Presentiment of Non-Being

Especially the *Four Prose Pieces* and "Obsequies" reveal Van Ostaijen's mode of phenomenological perception. "Lines" (from *Four Prose Pieces*) is a good example of this centripetal vision, of what Bachelard calls "se rêver a l'intérieur des choses." The *poëma* (III, 252) follows Heidegger's degrees of perception or knowing, since for Heidegger to know is to see; a formulation based on his etymology of the Greek verb ὁράω ("to see") being the root verb for εἶδος or ἰδέα, commonly translated as "idea." In

"Lines" Van Ostaijen wants to reveal that existence harbors extinction. He will show this in such a common occurrence as a middle-aged man walking down the street. The concrete man, (Mr. So and So) is put into parentheses to obtain the "Umkreis von Offenbarkeit," where the perception of his walking can manifest itself as a phenomenon. Now follows the *Freilegung*, the uncovering or laying bare of what this walking contains as essential importance. In the "as yet ordinary gait of this man lives the old man's walk."

The *Auslegung* makes this observation more explicit through a series of images. The man's "as yet normal gait" is like a "heavy ink line, but beneath it the other walk lies like a line of pale ink" wich "time will pull up" and the thick ink line "shall grow pale." The next image of the *Auslegung* is a curious usage in this context. Metamorphosis from chrysalis to imago is most often associated with the creative act: the caterpillar becoming the butterfly. But Van Ostaijen's interpretation of the chrysaline state is taken literally as a process of becoming and extinction. When the caterpillar sheds its cocoon and is transformed into a butterfly, it is in the process of dying. "Like a caterpillar in its cocoon, so the resilient young walk harbors the old one." Here again, Van Ostaijen unknowingly echoes Heidegger. For the German philosopher death "as an ontological characteristic of existence . . . is the possibility not to be." William Barrett summarizes this crucial issue of death in terms of Heidegger's phenomenological ontology as, "if my own possibility not to be is disclosed to me, this possibility becomes an actual constituent of my existence."[48] This is precisely the content and meaning of "Lines."

The images of the *Auslegung* all share the notion of erosion, fading away – all imply extinction. First the thick ink line which must give way, in time, to the pale one it covers over. Second, the cocoon, which, "when the time has come," cannot prevent the caterpillar from breaking through on its way to extinction. Third, the potential stoop of the old man hidden in "the smooth rectangle of his shoulders" is "like a circle which one might have drawn inside a square and then removed with an eraser." The fourth image is the most graphic and strongest of the series in discovering extinction as a hidden potential in this man in the prime of his life. Once the other three images have made you *see* "that the ordinary man walking there is losing his sturdy outline," you are prepared to see this relentless change as that of "a sheet of paper which, thrown into the fire, shrinks in baroque curls toward the kernel of its ashes." Now one is prepared to accept this ontological possibility not to be. "You know now that you are still in the time of the unpierced hull. But you do not know or you forget that the caterpillar has already been living for a long time within the tissue." The caterpillar has become a symbol of death. And all the fear of extinction, despite the acceptance of its inevitability, is concentrated in the last, short line, which gives the *poëma* the *Unheimlichkeit* Hadermann speaks of: "Now and then it moves."

Who is the second person singular to whom the author addresses himself? He reoccurs in the other three *poëmata* of *Four Prose Pieces*. Jakobson notes that "besides the author and the reader, there is the 'I' of the lyrical hero or of the fictitious storyteller and the 'you' or 'thou' of the alleged addressee of dramatic monologues, supplications, and epistles." The *you* of these *poëmata* is an "alleged addressee," for it is no one else but Van Ostaijen himself. These *poëmata* are lyrical monologues addressed to himself. "Virtually any poetic message is a quasi-quoted discourse," states Jakobson.[49] Usage of the pseudo-addressee *you* is a technical method to allow Van Ostaijen to dream himself "a l'intérieur des choses." In this particular case it is also a means of disclosing to himself (as William Barrett puts it) the "ontological characteristic of existence . . . the possibility not to be." The term *disclosure* might summarize the phenomenological mode of perception: revealing to oneself the essences of phenomena. As Thévenaz was quoted before, phenomenology is "an adventure of consciousness" not a system. "It is a disclosure of phenomena, but at the same time it is a return to the self or to the subject. It aims at essences, and it ends up in existence." This phenomenological movement is the movement of these *poëmata*. Van Ostaijen seeks for the foundation of being in disclosing the essence of objects or phenomena: his poetic transcendentalism. But in all these pieces he returns to himself, to his own authentic existence.

To see is to know. Such a phrase would adequately sum up phenomenology's method, especially in the case of Heidegger. The first phrase of "Lines" clearly differentiates between mere physical seeing and the phenomenological mode of vision, an analogy to Kandinsky's physical and psychic values of colors. The *poëma* states at the beginning a normal act of vision: "You see a man in the street; he is not yet old, around fifty." But the author immediately states his amazement that there is something profoundly more to this man than his mere presence in the street. "For what you now suddenly see and at which you are amazed, you should have seen earlier, you should have seen just now, it is always present." The man is "bracketed," and the revelation comes from concentrating on the phenomenon of "how in this man's as yet normal gait lives the old man's walk." The rest of "Lines" is what Heidegger calls a *Zurückfragen* to the fundamental meaning of what that amazement constituted: that being

harbors non-being. This *Zurückfragen* by Heidegger to the fundamental
foundation of being leads, as in Van Ostaijen's "Lines," to "an ontology of
non-being, into a méontologie." The process by which this ontological
fact is established is the process of perception. In this short *poëma,* the
verb *to see* is used ten times. What this perception reveals is strange, but
true, and is essentially a simple act of stepping back "pour voir jaillir les transcendances" as Merleau-Ponty puts it. Merleau-Ponty continues to say that
this perception of the world will reveal it as "étrange et paradoxal." For
the act of knowing can be a paradoxical one: knowledge that the gait of a
man reveals inevitable extinction, that the emergence of the caterpillar
from his cocoon is the onset of death.

On the surface it might appear that "Lines" is a less prominent example
of metonymic art. However, Jakobson wisely cautions that in poetry there
are no absolutes. "In poetry not only the phonological sequence but in the
same way any sequence of semantic units strives to build an equation.
Similarity superimposed on contiguity imparts poetry its throughgoing [sic]
symbolic, multiplex, polysemantic essence . . . Said more technically, anything sequent is a simile. In poetry where similarity is superinduced upon
contiguity, any metonymy is slightly metaphorical and any metaphor has a
metonymical tint." [50] This is precisely the case in "Lines." The "normal
gait" becomes a metonymy for a) 'a man in the street," and b) existence.
Similarly, the "forward curving" of the man's straight shoulders is a metonomy for old age. The series of sequential imagery units build toward the
total effect of an equation: non-being resides in being. But the progression
of the images is a contiguous one. The initial theme of the walk of the old
man residing in the normal gait calls into being, through the process of
association (Van Ostaijen), contiguity (Jakobson), or *retentissement* (Bachelard) the series of images, a process similar to Van Ostaijen's *lyrisme à
theme.* Hence the thick and pale ink lines, the caterpillar in his cocoon, the
erased circle in the square, the sheet of paper curling to ashes are all metaphors for the walk of the old man residing in the as yet normal gait of
this man, but metaphors with a very definite "metonymical tint." Together,
as a "sequence of semantic units" striving "to build an equation," they
have the character of a simile. Since Van Ostaijen is essentially talking
about his own existence (the images of essences end up in existence), these
images function metonymically, in Jakobson's phrase, as "angrenzende
Widerspiegelungen, als metonymische Ausdrücke des Dichters Ich."

The images are also synecdochic expressions of being harboring non-
being. "Lines" is a good example of the two main characteristics of metonymic art according to Jakobson's theory: "die gegenseitige Durchdrin-

gung der Gegenstände (die Realisierung der Metonymie im eigentlichen Sinne) und ihre Zersetzung (die Realisierung der Synekdoche)..." The arbitrary sequence of the images – one could have come before the other, or vice versa – becomes a causal sequence, an autonomous *Verbindung*. "Der Dichter definiert die Kunst als gegenseitige Ersetzbarkeit der Bilder. Beliebige Bilder bergen nicht nur Ähnlichkeit und können folgliche gegenseitige Metaphern sein ... die beliebigen sind so oder so in der Möglichkeit benachbart." Undoubtedly "Lines" is an example of contiguous images being drawn together by a metonymical case of elective affinities. As a phenomenological *poëma*, or as a metonymic structure, "Lines" describes Van Ostaijen's awakening to the reality of the inevitable ontological affinities of death and life.

A remarkable parallel to "Lines" is the last poem Van Ostaijen presumably wrote. "The Old Man" ("De Oude Man") also treats the theme of death hiding in existence. (II, 244)

An old man in the street
his brief story to the old woman
it is nothing it sounds like an empty tragedy
his voice is white
it is like a knife which was whetted so long
till the steel became thin
Like a utensil outside him hangs this voice
above the long black coat
The old skinny man in his black coat
is like a black plant
See you this gasps through your mouth
the first taste of a narcosis

One could interpret this poem as an extension (its limit) of "Lines." Now the man "around fifty" of "Lines" is an "old man in the street." His life has been completely reduced to the barest form of existence; it has become a "brief story," "nothing," an "empty tragedy." His voice has been reduced to a colorless "white" and as thin (i.e., barely audible, barely existing) as a knife honed to the thinnest of edges. Notice how the old man himself is bracketed to concentrate on his voice, just as in "Lines" Van Ostaijen concentrated on the phenomenon of the walk to pierce through to the profundity of existence. A series of three images about the old man's voice progresses contiguously, very much in the same manner as the images of the walk in "Lines." "Story" evokes "nothing," and "empty tragedy" recalls "voice." The preceding negative adjectives "brief," "nothing," and "empty" build to the full force of the image: "his voice is white." Though technically the triple use of "is like" classifies the images in this poem as similes, they appear to be again a case of Jakobson's "similarity super-imposed on contiguity."

The poem is divided into two equal parts, with the seventh verse as dividing line. This verse once more reiterates the barely existing phe-nomenon of the old man's voice with the (almost brute) force of "utensil." The voice is now no longer even a part of the man, but is so useless that it appears to be separated from him, a utility, and no longer inextricably commingled with the man's total organic existence. Thus, the second half of the poem proceeds contiguously to reunite the synecdochic "voice" with the man's existence as a final statement of complete uselessness. The triple repetition of "black" in the second half enforces this sense of doom, as opposed to the single use of "white" in the first half. The "old skinny man" is inside "his black coat" like a shriveled larva inside the dead hull of his cocoon. Not only does he lead an extreme of reduced existence, a vege-table life, but he leads it as a rotted plant which, though still holding up, is really already dead.

The second to last verse has the same use of *you* as in "Lines." The essence of this old man, death, is returned to the subject of the poem, the author's consciousness. But here it is no longer, as in "Lines," the *possi-bility* of non-being, but the realization of the fact of death itself. Again the phenomenological use of the verb of vision has distilled the essences of the phenomenon of the old man (his voice, his black coat) to make the author (*you*) know the fact of his own potential death. The existential fear is no longer a paradoxical strangeness, but a simple confession of this fear; "See you this gasps through your mouth / the first taste of a narcosis." Natural-ly, the last word is not only anaesthesia's artificially induced extinction, but also life's narcosis of old age: the onset of death. "Lines" and "The Old Man" are but two examples of the close resemblance in method and con-tent of Van Ostaijen's final lyrics and the prose pieces written after the major grotesques.

"Nicolas": Fearful Recognition of Non-Being

"Nicolas" (III, 250–251), more cryptic than "Lines," is a variation on the same theme of a search for the fundaments of being, which leads to a formulation of non-being. Though the *poëma* opens like a fairy tale, it soon develops into a description of a crisis of identity, which in turn deepens into the fundamental question of life and death. The "argument" of "Nicolas" is quite simple. Nicolas is a man without a last name, or at least, no one knows him by any other but his first. This fact sets him apart from other people. The barber, for example, as well as acquaintances do not address him in the normal fashion, but separate him from others in even such a simple act as greeting customers in a barber shop. "It happens sometimes that an old customer enters after Mr. Nicolas, and he greets: Hello, everybody, hello, Mr. Nicolas."

In European society the social code is much stricter about the formality of first and last names. To have everyone, even people below his station in life such as the barber, the apprentice barber, the maid, even the parrot in the barber's shop, call him by his first name would lead more easily to feelings of inferiority than it might in America. In other words, he is not considered to be like other people. Furthermore, the emphasis on the first name concentrates more on the individual person. A first name is more intimately related to someone than a family name, the species instead of the genus. Being always called by his first name, Nicolas is constantly reminded of himself as an individual, rather than as a more anonymous entity, Mr. So and So. How important socially one's name can be was demonstrated before by Van Ostaijen in the little grotesque "A Fatality" ("Een fataliteit"), where a man is also extremely sensitive to his (ludicrous) name. (III, 330–331) Curiously enough, this little tale also starts with the typical fairy-tale introduction but it remains a social satire. Though this distinction between first and last name might seem fatuous, Van Ostaijen takes great pains, considering the length of the *poëma,* to establish this fact and to hint at its disturbing influence on Mr. Nicolas.

The second immediate question is: why the name Nicolas? The Biblical allusion would suggest the Nicolas in the New Testament who was chosen as one of the Seven to spread the Gospel among the Greek-speaking Jews (Acts, 6 : 5). There is no other Nicolas in the Bible, and of this man little is known beyond the fact that he was considered a "proselyte," i.e., a convert to Judaism, someone who is essentially a stranger to the faith. The obscurity of this New Testament figure, though of such importance as a minister of the Gospel, might be the basis for the strange dream of wish-fulfilment, couched in Biblical terms of a visitation of God to a new prophet (= one who *reveals* the word of God): the non-existing prophet Nicolas. "Once again there will come a prophet. He will be awakened in the middle of the night and the voice of Elohim shall call and the vowels shall surely ricochet: 'Nicolas, Nicolas! Have you heard my voice, Nicolas!'" The implication is, of course, a negative one. There will be no prophet Nicolas who would give his name stature lasting across centuries. For Nicolas is not a hero, not even a hero "of a novel by Restif de la

Bretonne." [51] He will never make true the claim of what his name literally means, "conqueror of the people," he will always be merely Mr. Nicolas. After this long preamble (three-fourths of the piece), Van Ostaijen concentrates on the major issue, what or who is this Nicolas.

As in "Lines," a process of reduction seems to have been taking place. First, Nicolas is introduced as quite ordinary, no hero, not even in a novel by Restif de la Bretonne. The absence of a family name sets him apart socially. Nicolas becomes somewhat ridiculous by the socially diminishing iteration of his name. Secondly, his name is used by the maid to lie about his presence to a friend, who happened to drop by in the evening. The reduction has become more important, becomes closer associated with Mr. Nicolas himself, musing alone in his room. *Lie* is used twice in quick succession. His absence was a lie. But it is his name which assumes the proportions of that lie. "How heavy weighs such a lie with the bright vowels and the stress on the last syllable on one's conscience. For every time the stress is like a hammerblow which drives the nail deeper in the receding mass of conscience, built on the lose sand of a lie, Nicolas!" Clearly, the second lie is not a social ruse to preserve his privacy, but is the name itself. A brief stop to the reduction is the wishful dream of becoming a prophet chosen by Elohim for the task of fame, then the final reduction brackets even the name itself. Nicolas is no longer Nicolas, but "this name worse than a name and worse than a shadow" – Nicolas himself as a living reality harboring his own extinction. Nicolas has become a lie unto himself, sensing that he is excluding a very important and profoundly fearful aspect of himself.

The fear of the last paragraph of the *poëma* is hinted at in the repeated "stress on the last syllable" of his name. In such a scrupulous craftsman as Van Ostaijen, such details are significant. *Las,* the last syllable of his name, in French means "tired," "weary," or even "disgusted." Mr. Nicolas is tired of the lie of his name, tired of the lie of himself, but not yet willing to admit what he is afraid of disclosing to himself. To penetrate the secret of his name, Nicolas takes a similar step of distancing (bracketing) as the author did in "Lines." The last paragraph takes place within the consciousness of Nicolas himself who, as in a dramatic monologue, addresses himself in the second person singular. By putting himself in parentheses, which allows him to look upon himself as a phenomenon, the phenomenon of "this name," he is able through the process of *Zurückfragen* to lay bare that which was hidden to him. His own name has been bracketed, and is now no more than a phenomenon of "bright vowels." The reduction is complete. Nicolas has dreamed himself (the scene hints at a dark room in the evening) into the phenomenon of his name, leading him to the foundation of his existence, and to fear. What he will find is kept suspended to the very last set of phrases. It is again a process of illumination, of seeing which is knowing; "for now you see, by the lantern of these vowels, your darkness and that there are corners, so black, that the most tried tactile sense shivers and hides."

An intricate web of images, this final paragraph weaves abstracted, metonymic representations of the major *Absonderung* ("this name" or "those bright vowels" instead of *Nicolas*) into an example of Jakobson's *Berührungsassoziation,* until the final revelation has been reached. When his name is put into parentheses, Nicolas looks at it as merely a name, only to have to admit its accompanying shadow. The metonymy has been called into independent existence, and "die Äusserung des Gegenstandes nimmt auf sich seine Funktion." A similar process as that in "Lines" has occurred. *Nicolas* as a name, has become a) "this name worse than a name and worse than a shadow," b) its shadow, c) "those bright vowels." The crucial image is that of the shadow. His name having a shadow is similar to the image in "Lines" of the thick ink line and its corresponding pale one underneath it, or the erased circle in the square; it is the presence of non-being in being, extinction within the reality of his name. One could, perhaps, take the shadow most simply to mean death. The revelation, the uncovering of *das Verborgene* ("for now you see"), is the acceptance of the shadow, and of the name "which has the power of the shadow and like a shadow who can cry." Paradoxically, understanding the meaning of the shadow and accepting its presence as the shadow of his name will bring understanding; shadow will bring light ("for now you see, by the lantern of these vowels, your darkness"). Nicolas is discovering for himself what Merleau-Ponty describes as the essential value of shadow: "L'ombre ne devient ombre . . . que lorsqu'elle cesse d'être devant nous comme quelque chose a voir, et qu'elle nous enveloppe, qu'elle devient notre milieu, que nous nous y établissons." (PP, 358) Or, as William Barrett sums up Heidegger's phenomenological reduction of ontology to méontology, Nicolas, through accepting the presence of his name's shadow, must accept the "ontological characteristic of existence . . . the possibility not to be."

But the fear of this truth is terrifying. "That's why you're so terribly afraid." He still tries to negate or ignore its existence. "And you keep silent since you hope that it too will be silent, the shadow." But it will not keep silent; Nicolas has to admit its existence, has to admit that his name, the phonemic label of his authentic existence, has its shadow of death. Hence the mere uttering of his name is sufficient to call up this dreadful fact.

"You hear: 'Good evening, Mr. Nicolas.'" That is sufficient, terror strikes: "and before you have looked past the steam of your fear . . ." This image, as well as some others in this final paragraph of "Nicolas," illustrate Jakobson's theory of how the metonymic abstraction takes on autonomous existence as a personification, assumes a synecdochic reality at the price of catachresis. There is his fear which issues "steam." The shadow which is not even merely an opposite of light, but the shadow of a name, assumes independent existence; it can cry out and it speaks. There is enough ambiguity, Jakobson's "similarity superinduced on contiguity," in the phrasing of the greeting at night, so that it can either be the shadow of his name greeting Nicolas or a fleeting recollection of such an actual occurrence, trivial in itself. His name becomes the phonemic triad of /i/, /o/, /a/, which in turn become independent objects of sound that "roll from terrace to terrace in your conscience," gaining in brightness until they become a "lantern."

The "bright vowels," the phonemic triad, sound ever deeper into Nicolas' consciousness, until he realizes that the name itself is not terrible, but that the sound of his name reveals the terrifying essence of his being. Perhaps nowhere else in these *poëmata* does Van Ostaijen state so clearly the phenomenological process of revealing that which was hidden than in the phrase that the vowels, the synecdoche for the name Nicolas, have "the clarity which depth hangs around the things that already carry their own limpidity . . ." Phenomena have their own essences, which need to be rediscovered. Husserl stated a *Selbstgebung* of the object or, as Thévenaz puts it: "The object is not *constructed* by this consciousness; it gives itself to the view of this consciousness." The vowels have their own phenomenological clarity; the vowels imply the same clarity for the name Nicolas as for the man who carries that name. Through the retrogressive action from vowel-triad to name to his own existence, Nicolas discovers what is "terrible," that the "shadow" of his name is the shadow of his life. Life is contoured by the shadow line of death. The cryptic complexity of these images, when "any metonymy is slightly metaphorical and any metaphor has a metonymical tint," is permissible in metonymic art with its reciprocal replaceability of images. Despite the multiplexity of metonymic art, the phenomenological venture of awakening to an essential ontological truth can be discerned. Nicolas has finally reached the fearful knowledge that his existence harbors his death; "for now you see, by the lantern of these vowels [his name], your darkness [his potential non-being], and that there are corners, so black that the most tried tactile sense shivers and hides."

"Nicolas" and "Lines" are *poëmata* that describe the adventure of consciousness to discover the foundation of being, which in turn discloses the inescapable truth of a corresponding *méontologie.* "Nicolas," too, has obvious similarities with the poem "An Old Man." Just as the old man is bracketed to rediscover him through the phenomenon of his voice, so Nicolas is bracketed by the concentration on "those bright vowels" of his name which, upon discovery of their essential meaning, lead back to his own existence. Indeed, the discovery of the immanence of death within the thick of being appears to be the central theme of these *poëmata,* as well as in a number of Van Ostaijen's most important final lyrics. Even in his purest lyrics one senses a nostalgia, a regret that the perfection of a natural phenomenon cannot be attained by human beings; a phenomenon, outside of man, does not have the capacity of knowing the fact of its ultimate extinction.

"Obsequies": Acceptance of Non-Being

"Obsequies" (III, 398) is the final variation on this fundamental theme. "Obsequies" is not one of the *Four Prose Pieces,* though it appears to belong to the same date of origin as these *poëmata.* In this *poëma* the theme of death is already stated in the title. Temporally it is divided into two parts, the first half takes place in the morning, the second in the afternoon. In the morning the poet describes the sensation of knowing autumn's presence in an August day. Van Ostaijen was particularly sensitive to these subtle changes in weather, when one season harbors a subsequent one. In "Small Forest," the first half of the *poëma* describes the presence of summer in spring, and in "O Thou, My Splendid Solitude," he senses the vernal season in March. These are but variations on one major theme in these *poëmata,* the ambiguity of existence, its inchoate quality which is connected with the presence of non-existence in the midst of a plenitude of being. All these *poëmata* are linked by this central cognition: the seasonal changes just mentioned, the thick ink line and its correlative pale one in "Lines," the three vowels and their shadow of the name "Nicolas," the presence of darkness in light as in "Obsequies" and "O Thou, My Splendid Solitude." This corresponds to Bachelard's "le *contre* et le *dans*" of images, Merleau-Ponty's essential ambiguity of existence, where meaning is "mixed up with non-meaning," and Heidegger's ontology revealing a méontology.

The opening paragraph of "Obsequies" is again an example of metonymic *Berührungsassoziation,* in which temporal sequences are reshuffled to fit the poet's vision, an individual contiguity becomes a causal sequence, and again there is the application of the central feature of Jakobson's metonymic art, the reciprocal replaceability of images. During a morning in

"mid-August" when it is "not hot, but mild, without being cool," the poet
senses the presence of "the September day, when summer really decomposes." The major theme has already been implied. With a sudden shift
peculiar to metonymic art, this fairly general observation of a seasonal
phenomenon, though extremely subtle, is relegated to one's own consciousness of existence. In the middle of August, one sees in the mind's eye the
September day and its effects, not only seasonal, but also organic: "when it
happens in front of our eyes and in our organs that the elements of summer separate." Realistically we can "not say of this mild day in August
that autumn is already visibly present in it," but a poetic phenomenology
of ontology can discern even here the thick ink line giving way tot the pale
one, for "we are like animals which, long before death, already smell decomposition." The sequence of images from "Lines" continues, now joined
by the image of the simultaneity of shadow and light first mentioned in
"Nicolas."

The *poëma* is progressing in time towards noon and, when the theme of
death is remembered, even such a simple observation as the precedence of
light over shadow on a street when the sun is almost at full strength, becomes a profound image. "Around eleven in the morning the sun has taken
much away from the street"; i.e., light has taken many shadows away,
darkness is hardly present in the street along which the poet is walking towards the ceremony of burial. Light is life and noon is the time of its
triumph; "we walk, almost more easily and surely more freely, on the
sunny side." And yet, the grievous occasion and the ever-present ambivalence of light and shadow cannot be ignored, for there are, nevertheless,
"spots where here and there the shadow still is." One unwittingly makes
the choice of walking in the sun rather than in the shadowy spots, a choice
made by the sad occasion.

The first paragraph gives the setting, the occasion, the subject, as well as
the time sequence of the *poëma*. An intermittent sentence, conjoining first
and second halves, states the central problem which will be resolved in the
final sentence. "And we feel now that there is nothing contradictory, without, however, being able to define the feeling precisely, between this mild
August day and the obsequies, which one is called upon to attend in yonder
church." In this calm, sober statement lies the crucial preoccupation with
life and death; but the anguish of "Nicolas" and the foreboding of "Lines"
have now been resolved in the acceptance of this fact. One should feel a
contradiction between the mournful occasion and the bright summer's day,
between light and darkness, between life and death. But there is precisely
no contradiction because both are one, the fullness of "le *contre* et le

dans." In "Obsequies" Van Ostaijen seems to have finally accepted Merleau-Ponty's "nous sommes toujours dans le plein, dans l'être," where "nothing" is just as expressive as "something," where "le silence est encore une modalité du monde sonore." The second half elaborates this theme. Most of these *poëmata* seem to follow a definite pattern. First, the naming of the object, which will be scrutinized in a phenomenological manner later on. Secondly, the premonition of a potential profundity, which stirs the poet's consciousness. Thirdly, the bracketing of the object and replacing it by a synecdochic detail, which will lead to the discovery of the phenomenon's essence. And finally, the return to one's existence, now seen in the different light of the ontological discovery. "Obsequies" is even more carefully divided. The first half, consisting of one paragraph, is separated from the second by a bridging sentence that refers back to the first and points forward to the second half, which is also one paragraph long. The final sentence, the coda, fulfills or sums up the "argument" of the intermediary sentence.

In the second half the procession has reached the church. The church, as a phenomenon, pays little attention to its symbolic role, but lies basking in the light of the sun; "such clarity one would be inclined to hold unusual in a church." The theme of contradiction is repeated throughout this section. Though such an observation might be "unusual," an improper reaction against social conditioning, one does not find it abnormal; "one finds it quite normal that [the light is] everywhere [very bright] save a few slanted shadows in the aisles." The latter addition iterates the "spots of shadow" on the almost noonday street of that morning. The repetition serves as connection. For the sentence, which immediately follows, opens with, "What one already brought along this morning . . ." The "what" is the presence of "the September day" in "mid-August," is sun and shadow, is the knowledge that life precludes the possibility of not being. That morning's message hinted at in phenomena, becomes now, during the funeral service in the church, "clear experience."

Conventions connected with such grave occasions as the present one no longer have the force to "order phenomena" according to what one is supposed to feel in terms of society. The knowledge of the inevitable commingling of life and death, now apprehended as an individual authentic experience, supersedes all conventions; "the notion of death as bitter finality against this experience of equable light, commands no longer this synthetic power, which, in us, could formerly order the phenomena according to this accompanying notion." "It is totally different." Indeed it is, for death is no longer a "bitter finality" but already present in existence,

just as light precludes darkness. The somber idea of the total finality of
death contrasts sharply with the light in the church, which reminds the
author of the knowledge "brought along this morning." "Two values stand
suddenly next to each other: death and light and we no longer succeed, as
before, to think the phenomena of this notion according to the order of the
other one." The realization has come that one cannot place one set of
values, those of death, *against* the other, those of light or life.

Previously Van Ostaijen used the metaphor, contrasting these still incongruous values, of a cork which "bobs on the water's surface." This
image of reaction, of opposing forces, is no longer valid. Instead "the flood
of light washes the cork constantly to the beach," a constant reciprocal
motion, which gives precedence to neither the cork nor the water. The
cork, from the previous context, is associated with the false notion of
death as a "bitter finality" of life, which comes suddenly and unexpected.
The water is apparently associated with the light, with existence. The
movement of the cork bobbing on the water's surface is the metaphoric
representation of the inextricable commingling of life and death, which
maintains the ambiguity of authentic existence. The motion of cork on
water recalls Merleau-Ponty's inchoate quality of the phenomenological
investigation, which is not a defeat of the method, but essential to the basic
meaning of "le mystère du monde et le mystère de la raison." Here the
note of continuity, noticed before in "Lines" or in "Strange Attack," is
present again.

The final sentence of the *poëma* describes Merleau-Ponty's wonder of
the phenomenological venture to find the essence of objects. By setting this
final sentence aside from the preceding paragraph, Van Ostaijen seems to
follow Merleau-Ponty's description and appears to "prend recul pour voir
jaillir les transcendances." The adverb which opens the sentence testifies to
the impact of the revelation. "Suddenly one stands with the accompanying
value-judgment of death as with a telescope in a room." The realization of
life harboring death has opened up the horizon of the author's consciousness, suddenly discarded the narrow confines of socially induced value-
judgments, and allowed him to see the infinitely more profound quality of
the ontological fundaments of being. A line of progressive states of knowledge links "Lines" to "Nicolas" and to "Obsequies." First in "Lines" the
realization and the foreboding quality of this revelation, which turns into
fear in "Nicolas," while finally in "Obsequies" this knowledge is accepted
and judged to be beneficial rather than fearful. "Obsequies" has a tone of
wonder and peace which is lacking in both "Lines" and "Nicolas."
It has the quality of a meditation and lacks the putting into parentheses

of the author as concrete man, in order to gain the necessary distance from himself. Van Ostaijen in "Obsequies" has attained Husserl's "essential intentional contact between consciousness and the world." The ontological reduction towards a *méontologie* has become a reality and a transcendental revelation.

"O Thou, My Splendid Solitude":
The Fullness of Being

"O Thou, My Splendid Solitude" (III, 253) seems to have as its text Merleau-Ponty's central thesis of man's fullness in his inextricable relationship with the world. "Nous sommes toujours dans le plein, dans l'être, comme un visage, même au repos, même mort, est toujours condamné à exprimer quelque chose . . . et comme le silence est encore un modalité du monde sonore." Man being always in his fullness even while in a state of suspension, like a person asleep, is substituted in Van Ostaijen's *poëma* by "aimlessness," and the phrase might be read: we are always in fullness, in being, even when in a state of aimlessness. During the "first vernal evening of March," the poet is sitting in a park in the evening, unhampered by trivial intrusions of ordinary existence, having released all conscious controls. It is a state of reverie when "aimlessness becomes the aim and settles with such forthrightness in the will, in a way that one so rarely – o this rarity of the enduring consciousness – observes in oneself." In its tone of peaceful meditation (which shows a phenomenological awareness of ontology), with its increased lucidity of vision (while dreaming oneself "à l'intérieur des choses"), "O Thou, My Splendid Solitude" shares the equable state of mind of "Obsequies." The fulsome praise of "o this rarity of the enduring consciousness" is lacking in the *Unheimlichkeit* of "Lines" and in the dread of "Nicolas."

The reflective dialogue form has returned. Here it seems to serve the purpose of musing to oneself, to keep the consciousness aware of the unfolding of phenomena, as if it were prone to fall into complete silence in this state of inactivity. Van Ostaijen reminds himself almost forcibly of his exact location, described in the first paragraph, which he invokes by typical contiguity of metonymic art. The word "therefore" hardly marks a rational conclusion; i.e., "aimlessness" as a state of mind hardly invites a rational causal relationship with a description of one's exact location, but in metonymic art even the most arbitrary contiguity can serve as causal sequence. The second paragraph describes Van Ostaijen's complete immersion into the world, the condition of Heidegger's *Dasein,* when one is exposed to "an area of revealibility, an area of opening up where something can manifest itself (as 'phenomenon')."[52] "One is glad, for one knows that this plenitude of aimlessness has its meaning in the rhythm of nature and that one, no matter how, can do nothing today which would not be part of it." The usually negative states of being or phenomena are replete with positive meaning for Van Ostaijen; "aimlessness" is plentiful and the lighted café is not needed in the "gathered darkness" of the evening, which is full of lucidity.

The next two paragraphs reveal how phenomenological consciousness is *weltlich* and how, in this state of Bachelard's *rêverie*, there is Husserl's *Selbstgebung* of phenomena. To obtain such an intimate revelation of being Van Ostaijen seems to have put, in Heidegger's phrase, the concrete man in parentheses, in order to allow his fulness of consciousness to absorb whatever phenomena happen to be present. First, there passes a bicyclist. Van Ostaijen displays again his extraordinary sensitivity to nuances. A bicyclist in winter and one in spring are quite different. "He has a light with a red glow and one does not quite know what he wants with this light in our darkness, which is vernal and can hardly bear the lamplight." Such a fine nuance of perception might seem trivial to some observers, but it is important, if only as revealing the state of mind of the author. This is a particularly fragile instance of Jakobson's dictum of metonymic art: "Zeige uns deine Umgebung, und ich sage dir, wer du bist." The *Umgebung,* in this instance, is this finely nuanced perception of the difference between a bicyclist's light in winter and in spring, and the promise of being able to locate the perceptor works retrogressively to the state of fulness of the author's plenitude of aimlessness.

In one other small piece, published posthumously, Van Ostaijen shows "this same hyper-sensitivity to barely perceptible nuances. "Biological Delimitation of the Dancer" ("Biologische begrenzing van de danser") states the simple fact that a professional dancer who performs in the Satyricon club and the same one who dances on his day off (Wednesday) in the Panthea club are not one and the same dancer. "So it happens that the Satyricon club on Wednesdays of every week counts one professional dancer less than on other days. The Panthea club, on the other hand, counts that day one more amateur dancer. It is a fine nuance, and one must have a great deal of practice in order to observe it." (III, 401) The latter, possibly tongue-in-cheek, observation is quite true in terms of Van Ostaijen's own poetic instances of this rare quality of perception. Certainly the *poëmata* under discussion testify to his acute perception.

Not only the bicyclist, but also people on foot pass by the poet, sitting on a bench in a park in his plenitude of aimlessness. The pedestrians are distinguished between strollers and people who just pass by. The first, the implication seems to be, are purposely "taking a stroll." There is a definite purpose, whatever the reason may be, to their evening walk. None have the aimlessness in their gait which would be more meaningful than the decisive act of choosing to take a stroll; none, the poet observes, pass by "just like that." Finally a Jewish family of four walks by and "scrutinize" the poet. Their glances "which slide across me" are not alike, but each has "its own specific light."

These four glances become one single one; an instance of metonymic art's predilection for an anthropomorphism "der unbeseelten Welt." Four glances, each distinctive, "with its own light" according to the individual, become "at my level" large and single; "finally *the* glance is past" and the single glance "remained insatisfied." That four glances become one and remain "unsatisfied" is the obverse of Van Ostaijen's perception, which would retain the fine nuances of each "own specific light," and be satisfied by the authenticity of individuality. The Jewish family cannot comprehend the purposeful aimlessness of someone who merely sits without choice, "on just any bench." This fact cannot be related to anything within their sphere of experience where everything must have a purpose and meaning. Yet the poet's aimlessness is more replete with meaning than their "meaningful" existence. This observation is corroborated by the end of the *poëma.*

There was one man who went by, just like that. The poet almost forgot him because the man did not pay him any attention, for "with sure steps he carried the same aimlessness with him." This man who "carried the same aimlessness with him" was freed by that fact from investigating whatever happened to his consciousness. He also knew that "splendid solitude" when phenomena "give themselves" to an open, aimless consciousness. "O Thou, my Splendid Solitude" is a *poëma* reminiscent of Husserl's phenomenological reduction, in which the "ensemble of all the empirical, rational, scientific judgments" have been bracketed in order to "bring to light this essential intentional contact between consciousness and the world." [53] This is a freedom which gives joy and a transcendental acuity of perception. Bachelard pointed out that this poetic "se rêver à l'intérieur des choses" (Husserl's *Selbstgebung*) is not a state of somnolence, but a stimulant of consciousness. "L'art est alors un redoublement de vie, une sorte d'émulation dans les surprises qui excitent notre conscience et l'empêche de somnoler." [54]

"Small Forest": The Phenomenon
of Light as Metonymic Art

Finally we return to "Small Forest," already discussed in terms of Kandin-sky's theory of colors. The entire first paragraph (the *poëma* consists of only two) can be seen as a final instance of metonymic art in these *poëmata* by Van Ostaijen. Again the factual 'subject' is simple: the difference in appearance of the pines of a small forest, between the time when it was seen in spring and now when seen at the beginning of summer. The ob-server, the author himself, is not a known factor. The images of the *Um-gebung* function as the metonymic expression of the poetic I. The experi-ence of the poetic I is one of wonder at a subtle change in the phenomena of the little pine forest. A fortnight ago it was familiar, now it has become "suddenly estranged and then, simply, strange." Temporal sequence is distorted, losing its normal causality for a causality of contiguity. "The sunbeams, so abruptly warmer from one day to the next and – we are in the month of June – for the first time warm and bright, have almost com-pletely prevented the possibility on the retina and in the brain of a relation-ship between the little forest of not very tall pines – there yesterday and saved in the memory – and this forest now, with the light, which is so total-ly different."

The agency of estrangement is the phenomenon of light. The sunbeams are metonymic expressions of a) the sun, b) the month of June, c) of light. The suddenness is brought about from the immediacy of conjoining tempo-rally separate parts of a sequence. "From one day to the next" means, in this case, from a fortnight ago *and* right now, which is immediately joined contiguously to the impossible possibility of the phenomenon of light on a pine forest as a reasonable factor (the brain) and a visual rationality (the retina). Yet it is so. It is precisely metonymic art which can best express the strange beauty, from a normal point of view, of a phenomeno-logical discovery of hitherto unperceived essences. The accidental beauty of the little forest under the uncertain vicissitudes of spring light is now a connective reality of light: "a structure of which the sunlight would be the mortar; indeed, from pine to pine and everywhere a gap could be, there is now the light, not as something accidental which could vanish, for instance when a cloud would push past the sun, no, but as a durable construction." In this sentence are various examples of Jakobson's *Berührungsassoziation:* whole to part (forest to pine), part to whole (pine to forest), cause to effect (beautiful events to chance), effect to cause (durable construction to light), spatial reference to temporal (the forest as a building to June), and the

Absonderung of established abstractions (the "mortar" of sunlight). Phenomenological perception realized through metonymic art, can now conclude the simple fact that "this is the relationship of the pines to each other and of the pines to the light."

But the concentrated force of this summer light, after the memory of the light of spring as something accidental, is too much for brain and retina to bear. One needs to find a counter-reality to restore a sense of equilibrium. This is achieved, as we saw before, in concentrating on the limiting, yet profound, color-sequence in the final paragraph. But before that chromatic harmony, both physical as well as psychical in terms of Kandinsky's theory, has been achieved, Van Ostaijen describes this "inordinate" quality of the light and its effects in a sequence of phrases which illustrate the power of metonymic art to create an independent verbal existence. The *Gegenstand* is this inordinate light, which is in turn *vergegenständlicht*. Accordingly, the creative metonymy transforms "die gewohnte Anordnung der Dinge." Proportions and distances between objects are changed to establish an autonomy of the "beliebige Kontiguität" with its "gegenseitige Ersetzbarkeit der Bilder."

The inordinate quality of the light becomes a metonymic reality; the inordinateness might stir the imagination of a prince to build himself a palace from this material. Rationality might interject with the observation that given the extraordinary quality of this light, why not a king instead of a prince, which would befit the rational sequence of superlatives? So Van Ostaijen interpolates "no not a king, but a prince such as Hamlet was a prince." "Die gewohnte Anordnung der Dinge" has been changed and a prince, though not any prince but its superlative (Hamlet), is superior to a king. The "beliebige Kontiguität" continues. The *Gegenstand* (bright sunlight), *vergegenständlicht* in "inordinateness," provides building-materials for a superlative prince, or for his parents, who want "to meet halfway the excesses of their deedless son and his insatiable satiety."

The sequential distance between a summer's day and the royal parents of a strange son is perfectly natural in the contiguity of metonymic art. This prince, described as an overreacher who can not satisfy his own demands, reminds one of Van Ostaijen's description of Hamlet, who for him is "the truth of the necessity of man's ultimate demise." The excess of this light can only halfway meet this prince's excesses. Now the prince is conjoined to the previous image of the retina. Arbitrary images not only have similarity, but can, as a result, be reciprocal metaphors, states Jakobson in his discussion of metonymic art. The superlative prince and the eye are similar and reciprocal metaphors; he becomes an eye "threadbare from the maddest realities of light." After this breaking point has been reached for the eye as well as for the prince, for the metaphor as well as for the author's reaction to this "inordinate" sunlight, only after this apex, can a return to establishing a balance be considered, only then can the prince have "peace of heart and tranquility of spirit." The last paragraph, as we saw before, performs precisely that task. The eye of the poet, and by implication the metaphoric prince, steadies and finds a beneficial soothing point of rest in the "motion of a brown hay wagon in the midst of the yellow-brown bed of needles." Brown signifies a return to an equable perspective, while the yellow remains as a connective to the joy of the experience of inordinate sunlight.

The grotesques played a sophisticated game with a world out of joint, and grimly asserted the futility of existence. These *poëmata* seem to be poetic testimony that Van Ostaijen's tempered pessimism about life's futility and the insufficiency of expression was perhaps not finally conquered, but was transformed into a profound acceptance of this fact. These prose pieces are in that sense optimistic. Van Ostaijen saw that "the lyrical emotion is a negation of a pessimistic view of life." Pessimism has been turned into a profound knowledge of the inevitability of life's darker side. The social world of the grotesques has been superseded by a metaphysical investigation of being and nothingness. Van Ostaijen discovered as his final lyrical task, the description of the joy in perceiving the essence of simple phenomena. During the final years of his life, Van Ostaijen appears to have withdrawn from the world of man to his private universe of lyricism. There he was both removed from the world as a social circus, and at the same time more deeply immersed in it as a structure of being. As these *poëmata* and his last lyrics show, he had finally found his true task, which happened to coincide with the program of phenomenology – to see the world of phenomena anew as the "freshly minted coin" of poetry. All Van Ostaijen finally asked for was his lyricism, to be "an ordinary poet." And the business of being simply a poet is to see the world as if newly created, unspoiled by the taint of man. This is what humbly, yet so profoundly, constitutes Van Ostaijen's mysticism.

APPENDICES

FOUR SHORT TALES

I. AQUARELLE

Aquarelle floats red. Blue and yellow. Around color bubbles swirls the water. In meeting the red and the blue become mild: mauve vibrates far up to the limit of experience. Wattmanpaper flows mauve-saturated. The mauve paper becomes grains of Wattmanpaper. Or: the yellow runs childlike desire towards the solution of stability. Blue rests, borders the vibration and determines the ratio inwardly: kernel. Children glint very long glitterapples.

The joy of stroking the paper wilts from my fingers. Fingers want to go further to the knowledge of my eyes. Desire: to feel the peace of blue and to penetrate to the limit of girl-childlike depth mauve vibration. Their wish is to be lips: quench, hands, thirst at the well of orange. This is the time of beauty for my fingers. Their total dissolution in their parasensual desire. They are no longer. They are only labile. They are becoming. Things which were fingers, now dissolved in the to be-eye-striving.

Until the eyes awaken, the dictators yearn for uprising. Poor fingers, idealists of the transferral of the spiritual to the parasensual. The eyes kill the things which dissolved themselves in the lability of too real desire. The fingers are fingers again. They were not that all of the time.

Poor fingers, each failure concludes the question: wherefore this desire to awaken from exactitude. Fingers were always fingers. They will never drink orange and never stroke mauve. Dictators do not like uprisings. It seems to me that sparkle-eyes cruelly chastise once bold fingers. Full of animal shame, thus my fingers hide their desire.

Perhaps it is just as well that the ultimate limit of my fingers is temporary hypertrophy of their desire. Perhaps it is just as well that eyes are dictators. And rebels weak.

Yet despite weakness it is rebellion. That my fingers were able to vibrate for a moment, briefly, in the delusion of being labile and on the way to realizing their desire.

II. ANAIS

That day the model Anais had received her monthly salary. She had postponed without effort every decision beyond this date. After short deliberation it was now clear to her how little change her salary could effect and, quickly associating, she concluded that it was not worth the trouble. One couldn't even consider an affair as a defense against boredom. Until the tram for which she had been waiting stopped, she had been dozing in the partial peace of suicidal contemplations. Then, with a graceful leap, she was in the car.

Pleasure for her: to recreate her leap mentally, in taut and lithe tailored lines. To realize that she felt better on the platform of the car than inside gave her a sense of self-sufficiency.

During the short ride to her place, she enjoyed the thought of throwing the money out of the window.

When she had taken her hat and jacket off, it had already become clear to her that throwing it away was no solution because the gesture itself was disproportionate. A few fifties and twenties float above the street, then eventually fall in such a manner that no one would notice them.

She found the idea silly, but just when she was going to relinquish it she was struck by the visualization of this act: thrifty banknotes over a street at twilight, the ordinary association scattered: this was, precisely, throwing money away.

Wrong: first to get the people, the shouting masses, interested through clowning and, after that, throwing the money by the bushel into the crowd – o the careful rule of the lavish scorner, to exchange the money for small change. The dissonance is clear between the psychic condition for this act – resignation – and the act itself – a positive rebellion with hope of salvation because of the rebellion.

This: twilight, you throw the few bills of your monthly salary out of the window. There are a few people on the street. No one notices the bills falling. Finally, and as an afterthought, the last bill, which lay long on the broad back of the wind, falls. You close the window, casually flip the switch and make light.

Anais thought immediately that it was now fitting not only to think the possibility through, as she did so often, but simultaneously to put thought into action. She took her handbag. Through the open window the wind threw a few short waves of freshness over her face and moist hands. Anais thought emphatically: I am young. And once again: I am young. It happened with the banknotes as she had imagined. Anais rested for a moment on the rare equilibrium between pondering and reality. Slowly the bills floated away from the window, took a seemingly brief upward direction, until several hung midway over the street. In the space – between the four story houses on each side – the street was a vacuum around the few bills. Anais followed them with her eyes, just as interested as someone can be who is suddenly surprised by the structure of a common object. Because she was familiar with the simple end of the last bill, which was still falling, she did not wait any longer at the window.

Alone in the room, she was uncertain. There remained a dissatisfaction in her like a slight nightmare. But her gesture had moved her such a distance from herself that she, laughing, observed that discontent was the only possible form of contentment for her.

III. CONVICTIONS

It happened that an accordion player, so confident in his skill and, as one is wont to say, so much at one with his instrument, not only pulled his instrument open as far as it would go but also, so to speak, as the superlative of this motion, tore his arm from his body. This procedure was naturally a mistake and the result of a momentary defect of consciousness. That is indeed the way to explain it.

To repair the damaging results of this mistake the aid of a doctor was required. And so a doctor was sent for. But this doctor – it appeared afterwards – was no less a man of conviction than the accordion player. He was very keen on being a good physician and, moreover, was keener still to hear people testifying to his being a good physician. Extremely touched by the unhappy incident and wholly intent on averting as soon as possible the most dangerous consequences of the disaster – so that everyone would congratulate him after the success for his skill as a physician – the doctor worked with such speed and absorption that only on finishing the treatment did he ascertain his colossal mistake. The mistake was that the doctor had joined the accordion instead of the arm to the body of the poor accordion player. Only when, in order to exhibit the affair as a clean and faultless job, he wanted to place the accordion in the hand of the accordion player, did he notice to his utter amazement – as one is also wont to say – that it was the arm that was left. He could not deny himself, however, the conviction that the arm and the accordion, from the point of view of causality, belonged to each other; from which it followed that, with the aid of a thin but strong piece of string, he tied the arm to the accordion.

Before departing he stroked the silk of his top-hat with his sleeve and naturally in the right direction – that is, with the silk. He then took his leave of the poor accordion player's wife, saying there was no reason to be dismayed.

IV. Curious Attack

Stabile he is madder. If he changes in such a way that instead of being he becomes becoming, he is carmine red. Such is he as soon as he moves.

He. The madder-carmine red. Not abstract: the madder. He is extremely concrete. Yet I would not be able to say in what manner he is concrete. Only, it seems to me: arching and oscillating on the perimeter-fragment. Movement is: to displace weight from left to right and to oscillate. He could be a very baroque dachshund whose paws disappear in the belly. Natural desire for unnaturalness. A whim.

While writing I realize how incorrect it would be to express: carmine red. Precisely the concrete is the bizarre entity of this deformation of nature according to laws of the purely conceivable. But it is also incorrect: the carmine red form. As such he is again too defined: concretely appearing abstraction.

Separated from the madder red by blue, opaline, mauve and manifold tremors of values lies the rose square. The rose square is peaceful. Subconscious cause of this is the delusion of the impermeability of the royal blue, the opaline and the values. The rose thinks: *he* can't touch me. First of all there is the royal blue which is indivisible in hardness, after that the impermeable force of the undulation of the opaline and the values. The rose square is at ease, therefore. And lies island-secure in values, the closest waves.

Then it happens. The madder rises up and sways on his arch. Exertion to oscillate. Presses immensely towards the right and becomes croplike malevolent when he notices the ungainliness of his organism and the objective peace of the rose at the other side of the royal blue.

Inarticulate fury sticks in his – the madder red – throat. The throat must be swollen. Only nothing indicates it. Where is the throat. The madder red is indeed only apparently archlike. The where of the organs remains unknowable in this baroque organism. What is knowable seems always the psychic cause for expression. Apparently unavailing and relationless to the result he becomes carmine red.

Perhaps because it would go faster, I lose sight for a moment of the carmine red. When I find him again, he has, wonder how, advanced near the royal blue. He attacks the royal blue. With the beak. Where is the beak. Probably were line and perimeter-fragment meet. Did I not think before that there was also the muscle-end of the organ of motion. Beak and motion-organ. It is unbelievable, could one mean just as well: such a structure is purely cerebral. Nevertheless: I see the action of the madder red. One cannot question its positive result. Much too clearly did I see the movement before, how he oscillated, and now the beak. Direct sharpbill in the compact clump of the royal blue.

The hardness of the royal blue greatly heightens the anger of the carmine red and, its inevitable result, his attack's sharpness. This happens suddenly: one half of the carmine red sticks right into the clump of the royal blue.

Now I seem to see the carmine red much clearer. He is completely mouth. I said already that the carmine red is probably archlike. Actively-organic he is always completely that organ which is just then functional. The carmine red is in turn as much as left leg, right leg, mouth. Thus the carmine red has no organs. He is always organ. One single organ. Becoming-in-action. Not in such a manner that the form changes. From the vantage point of his alternately becoming organs he is the transcendentally given. To me he is archlike. But this arch experiments functionally in a very strange, I would almost say, crazy manner. He has now, suddenly completely mouth, swallowed a large clump of the royal blue.

The opaline notices this. It shudders. So terribly terrified is the opaline that its spine – its more pronounced tones – weakens. These tones finally disappear in an indeterminateness like the milky way.

The carmine red oscillates. He grins. Cruelly satisfied hunger rouses hunger. The archform is an open mouth. Licks his chops right in front of his prey: the mauve.

The rose sees the danger. Dream befalls the miscalculation in the certainty of the unconditionally being separated.

The rose rises straight up. To drive strength to center, a moment, to conquer desperation. Then – the die is cast – the rose makes the leap into neighbouring values. The mauve guards the rear, the retreat. Balanced in the values the rose and the mauve dissolve.

The values vibrate. And are a little later again mirror-smooth rest. The carmine red winds up in the midst of the values. But the values are indeed impervious undulation. Where they become a hard resistance-proof mass, resilience compensates the lost ability of undulating. Hardened values evade the attack of the carmine red through a hard resilient leap – like a flea.

The carmine red is furious in the midst of this game-defense of the values. If they at least would defend themselves seriously. So nasty: while playing to escape the danger of being gobbled up. The carmine red oscillates mightly. The mouth becomes right leg again. Oscillation. Left right left. Left leg.

The carmine red is again madder.

FOUR PROSE PIECES

SMALL FOREST

After an acquaintanceship begun fourteen days earlier, this morning the little forest of not very tall pines became suddenly estranged and then, simply, strange. The sunbeams, so abruptly warmer from one day to the next and – we are in the month of June – for the first time warm and bright, have almost completely prevented the possibility on the retina and in the brain of a relationship between the little forest of not very tall pines – there yesterday and saved in the memory – and this forest now, with the light, which is so totally different. The difference is so great that, where yesterday you ascribed the most beautiful circumstances of this forest to chance, today you discern everywhere a connection, yes, a structure of which the sunlight would be the mortar; indeed, from pine to pine and everywhere a gap could be, there is now the light, not as something accidental which could vanish, for instance when a cloud would push past the sun, no, but as a durable construction. This is the relationship of the pines to each other and of the pines to the light. But there is something extravagant about it. So extravagant that you might think a prince – no, not a king, but a prince such as Hamlet was a prince – would have wanted a palace from such singular materials; or his parents might have wanted it: to meet halfway the excesses of their deedless son and his insatiable satiety. For they guessed that peace of heart and tranquillity of spirit could be his only after his retina became threadbare from the maddest realities of light.

You must lie on the ground. Thus, across the ground, past much ochre and brown, past much green, your eye gains the bark and again the green, the old and the young and finally this grey, this crazy grey-green, which is so exhausting that your eye flees to earth and slowly, only slowly, awakens to the motion of a brown hay wagon in the midst of the yellow-brown bed of needles.

NICOLAS

Once upon a time there was a man. His name was Nicolas and everyone called him by his Christian name: Mr. Nicolas. Allow me right away to explain that there is no resemblance between this Mr. Nicolas and the one who is the hero of a novel by Restif de la Bretonne. No, I do not mean a hero of any story, but a man who, be he no hero, is in all honesty called Nicolas and to whom one says: Mr. Nicolas. Now, one could think that this being called Nicolas, is neither terrible nor exceptional. I understand this point of view, but I do not share it. On the contrary. I do find it terrible and exceptional; I find it even terribly exceptional and exceptionally terrible. For when Nicolas enters the barbarshop, the barber says: "Good day Mr. Nicolas," and immediately following, without a pause be‑ tween, races the voice of the apprentice shrill after it: "Good day Mr. Nicolas"; and, as if one were at the bottom of a narrow valley where the echo is bounced back and forth, thus calls the parrot after the apprentice and the barber: "Good day Mr. Nicolas." It happens sometimes that an old customer enters after Mr. Nicolas, and he greets: "Hello, everybody. Hello, Mr. Nicolas."

Is he at home in the evening and he feels nice and cozy: alone with his wife and, for example, in the midst of memories of his youth ("Yes, that Harry Lam‑ merse, he was a damned nice fellow"), he suddenly hears the maid lie to some‑ one, probably a friend who just dropped by: "Mr. Nicolas is not at home. Mrs. Nicolas is not at home either. Yes, they are probably at the opera. Sure, tomorrow you have a good chance to catch Mr. Nicolas." How heavy weighs such a lie with the bright vowels and the stress on the last syllable on one's conscience. For every time the stress is like a hammerblow which drives the nail deeper in the receding mass of conscience, built on the loose sand of a lie, Nicolas! – Once again there will come a prophet. He will be awakened in the middle of the night and the voice of Elohim shall call and the vowels shall surely ricochet: "Nicolas! Nicolas! Have you heard my voice, Nicolas!"

For this name is worse than a name and worse than a shadow. It is like a name which has the power of the shadow and like a shadow who can cry. If you deal with such a shadow, you will never know whether you can trust its silence. That's why you're so terribly afraid. And you keep silent since you hope that it too will be silent, the shadow. But suddenly it is no longer silent. You hear: "Good evening, Mr. Nicolas." And before you have looked past the steam of your fear, the man who greeted is already far away. This is nothing. But that those bright vowels, spoken only once, sound from wall to wall and roll from terrace to terrace in your conscience, ever deeper, and that they furthermore have the clarity which depth hangs around the things which already carry their own limpidity, that is terrible: for now you see, by the lantern of these vowels, your darkness and that there are corners, so black, that the most tried tactile sense shivers and hides.

LINES

You see a man in the street; he is not yet old, around fifty. He seems ordinary. So he is. For what you now suddenly see and at which you are amazed, you should have seen earlier, you should have seen just now, it is always present.

That is, how in this man's as yet ordinary gait lives the old man's walk. You see the ordinary gait now like a heavy inkline, but beneath it the other walk lies like a line of pale ink and you know that time will darken this line when the other lightens. Like a caterpillar in its cocoon, so the resilient young walk harbors the old one. And nothing prevents the caterpillar from breaking through the cocoon, when the time comes.

And in the smooth rectangle of his shoulders you see a curving forward that is not visible to the naked eye and yet you see it. Like a circle one might have drawn inside a square and then removed with an eraser. The line disappeared, but the impression which the pencil made with the lead remains.

When you have seen this and the other, you see that the ordinary man walking there is losing his sturdy outline and that the contour of this man is changing perceptibly, just as a sheet of paper which, thrown into the fire, shrinks in baroque curls toward the kernel of its ashes.

With this man you saw how the hull was discarded and how his solidity is no different from the cocoon which hides the caterpillar from his presently old form.

You know now that you are still in the time of the unpierced hull. But you do not know or you forget that the caterpillar has already been living for a long time within the tissue.

Now and then it moves.

O Thou, my Splendid Solitude

This is the first vernal evening of March, no longer fresh but humid already, humid. Perhaps you know such an evening, experienced it in the same way I did: when aimlessness becomes the aim and settles with such forthrightness in the will, in a way that one so rarely – o this rarity of the enduring consciousness – observes in oneself. Therefore I am lured by this bench at the end of the lane, by the entrance to the park. You know: the lane which ends in a square behind which a woman stands high on a pedestal and she has a torch. She also leans heavily on one hip. It must have been a trying pose for the model. And there is the café at the left, where you leave the park and there is light.

Nevertheless, this is an evening when one loves the gathered darkness and places oneself in its midst with nothing but this full aimlessness. One is glad, for one knows that this plenitude of aimlessness has its meaning in the rhythm of nature and that one, no matter how, can do nothing today which would not be part of it.

There is a late bicylist. It can also happen in winter that you see a late bicylist. But this bicylist is now totally different. He has a light with a red glow and one doesn't quite know what he wants with this light in our darkness, which is vernal and can hardly bear the lamplight.

There are also some people passing by – among them merely casual strollers. All those passing by wonder why I, there by the entrance, merely sit on just any bench. It is strange that no one *just* passes by. Finally there is a Jewish family, who scrutinize me. In front walks the young man, the Jewish bridegroom, and next to him the Jewish bride. Then there is the old Jewess and the younger sister, obviously the sister of the bride. That makes four glances which slide across me, each with its own specific light; then they become, at my level, large, and finally the glance is past; but I do feel that something in it remained unsatisfied. The bridegroom was, of the whole bunch, the shyest.

I almost forgot one man who did just pass by without paying any attention to me. His face stood on a long neck, sharply forward and far from the trunk. He has not paid me my due.

With sure steps he carried the same aimlessness with him.

PROSE POEMS

The Sirens

Not so long ago sailors succeeded in catching the sirens, a few miles south of the Azores. The sirens whistled heartrendingly but the sailors, being literally deaf, remained unaffected. They wanted to purge the seas of these dangerous creatures and locked the sirens in a dark closed-off corner of the hold. In the harbors where their ship moored they were, after they had told of their catch, treated by seamen with jubilation and hurrahs and, since sailors believe that a captured siren is a talisman, they had no problem selling the sirens in Lisbon, Liverpool and Rotterdam; but only deaf sailors could lodge the sirens in the darkest corner of the ship's hold, the others knowing themselves unequal to the task.

Everyone knows that sea captains are people who want to use everything to their own advantage. So it was to be with the captured sirens. A round opening was made in the wall of the sirens' brig and from this opening a pipe carried the sirens' whistling far above the deck, above the sea, above the stream and the city. For the sirens to whistle when it seemed useful or pleasing to them, the seamen made a thin lance ending in three sharp needles. These needles were dipped in poppy juice and through a small opening in the brig were thrust into the body of the captured sirens. Poppy juice, when absorbed, produces an indescribable longing for space and an unlimited sadness. In sirens it awakens their past of distant seas, their former power over men and an ultimate sadness in which, as in another dimension, lie all of space and all delusions of power. Then the sirens scream very loudly; the endless vibrations of the whistling shoot sharply across the ship into space, suspended above the stream and the city. Seamen and people on shore say in the middle of their revels: it's twelve, the sirens whistled, the new year begins.

Yet, despite their captivity, the sirens have not relinquished their power. True, they are no longer able to entice blue jackets to the depths of the deep sea, where their song is an untimely death amidst the wonder of anemones and seaweed, shells and coral. But those who have once heard the whistling of the sirens high over the city, for the rest of their lives cannot suppress their longing for this lament. They have, like the mouse to the cat, fallen prey to the harbor, where they know the ships and the sirens.

Owners of factories in the country have bought sirens for their workers; they keep them captive in the cellars of their buildings. No matter what they try, they are not able to bring the sirens to make the plaintive wailing which these creatures aboard ship let out. One suspects that the sirens, lacking their ultimate pleasure, the smell of the sea, are slowly pining away. Besides, it is the water of the sea which gives their voices this sharpness.

OBSEQUIES

When, mid August, it is not hot, but mild, without being cool, we are not able any longer (as we were in June) to regard this temperature as a probable short, intermediary stage of which, according to the few experiences we have on this subject, the causes can be many and varied, but we do sense in this mildness, through our memory, the September day, when summer really decomposes, when it happens in front of our eyes and in our organs that the elements of summer separate. Hence we do not say of this mild day in August that autumn is already visibly present in it, no, but we are like animals which, long before death, already smell decomposition. Around eleven in the morning the sun has taken much away from the street and we walk, almost easier and certainly more losely, on the sunny side, rather than on the spots where here and there the shadow still is.

And we feel now that there is nothing contradictory, without, however, being able to define the feeling precisely, between this mild August day and the obsequies, which one is called upon to attend in yonder church.

The rural church lies stretched out in yon unsieved clarity. Such clarity one would be inclined to hold unusual in a church, but one does not: one finds it quite normal that it is very light everywhere, save a few slanted shadows in the aisles. What one already brought along this morning, becomes in this church a clear experience: the notion of death as bitter finality against this experience of equable light, commands no longer this synthetic power, which, in us, could formerly order the phenomena according to this accompanying notion. It is totally different. This notion of death bobs almost visibly against the clarity of the church, like a cork bobs on the water's surface. Two values stand suddenly next to each other: death and light and we no longer succeed, as before, to think the phenomena of this notion according to the order of the other one. But instead the flood of light washes the cork constantly to the beach.

Suddenly one stands with the accompanying value-judgment of death as with a telescope in a room.

CHRONOLOGY OF PAUL VAN OSTAIJEN'S CREATIVE PROSE *

1919

"Claire's Herd" ("De kudde van Claire")
(MS dated; publ. post.)

"Camembert"
(MS dated; publ. post.)

"Jus primae noctis"
(MS dated)

"Between Fire and Water" ("Tussen vuur en water")
(publ.)

"The General" ("De Generaal")
(MS dated; publ. post.)

"Portrait of a Young Maecenas" ("Portret van een jonge maeceen")
(conj.: Borgers in *Maatstaf*, X, No. 7 [October 1962], 431)

"Bankruptcy Jazz" ("De bankroet-jazz")
(Conj.: B 334)

1920

"The Marvelous Novel" ("De fijne roman")
(publ.)

"The Kept Hotel Key" ("De gehouden hotelsleutel")
(MS dated; publ. post.)

* This chronology is as accurate as are the given sources. A few dated manuscripts have been found (= MS dated). But for the majority only the date of publication is known (= publ.) or one has conjectured the year of origin (= conj.). A large number of pieces were published posthumously (= publ. post.). The bibliographical information, except where indicated, is from Gerrit Borgers' second, fully revised edition of the third volume of Van Ostaijen's *Collected Works*, which incorporates all the data which have come to light in the past decade: *Verzameld Werk. Proza I*, ed. G. Borgers, 2d. ed. (Den Haag, Antwerpen, 1966). References to this edition are noted as B, followed by the page number.

"The Conviction of Notary Telleke" ("De overtuiging van Notaris Telleke")
(publ.)

"The Man with the Head of a Swine" ("De man met de zwijnskop")
(conj.: B 343; publ. post.)

"Mechtildis, That Good Girl" ("Mechtildis, die goede meid")
(conj.: B 344; publ. post.)

"Colonialism" ("Koloniale politiek")
(conj.: B 344; publ. post.)

"Hierarchy" ("Hiërarchie")
(conj.: B 344; publ. post.)

"History" ("Geschiedenis")
(publ.)

1920–1921

"Intermezzo"
(conj.: B 346; publ. 1929)

"The Poet's Occupation" ("Het beroep van de dichter")
(conj.: B 345; publ. post.)

1921

"The Prison in Heaven" ("Het gevang in de hemel")
(publ.)

1923

"Work and Save" ("Werk en Spaar")
(publ.)

"The Money-Box" ("De cassette")
(publ.)

"Splendor and Decline of a Politician" ("Glans en verval van een politiek man")
(publ.)

"A Fatality" ("Een fataliteit")
(publ.)

"The Adventures of Mercurius" ("De lotgevallen van de Mercurius")
(publ.)

"City of Builders" ("De stad der opbouwers")
(publ.)

"The Fatal History of Scholem Weissbinder" ("De noodlottige geschiedenis van Scholem Weissbinder")
(publ.)

"Of a Windfall that was a Misfortune" ("Van een meevallertje dat een malheur was")
(publ.)

1924

To Be Pondered by Gentlemen Equestrians (*Tot overwegen voor hereruiters*)
(Van Ostaijen's Kafka translations. MS; epistolary evidence; publ. 1925)

Four Short Tales (*Vier korte vertellingen*)
(publ.)

1924–1925

Zoo for Children of Our Time (*Diergaarde voor kinderen van nu*)
(MS; epistolary evidence; publ. 1926)

"The Ash" ("De Es")
(conj.: B 329 + 349; publ. post.)

1925

"Patriotism Incorporated" ("De trust der vaderlandsliefde")
(publ.)

1926

"Ika Loch's Brothel" ("Het Bordeel van Ika Loch")
(publ.)

"Obsequies" ("De uitvaart")
(conj.: B 350; publ. post.)

"This Isn't Funny At All" ("Dit is helemaal niet geestig")
(conj.: cf. B 350; it appears to belong to the collection *Clew of Ariadne* published in 1928; publ. post.)

"Biological Delimination of the Dancer" ("Biologische begrenzing van de danser")
(conj.: cf. B 350; it appears to belong to the collection *Clew of Ariadne* published in 1928; publ. post.)

1927

Four Prose Pieces (*Vier Proza's*)
(MS; epistolary evidence; publ. 1928)

"The Lost House Key" ("De verloren huissleutel")
(publ.)

1928

Clew of Ariadne (Kluwen van Ariadne)
  (publ.)

1932

"The Gang of the Trunk" ("De Bende van de Stronk")
  (publ.)

BIBLIOGRAPHY

WORKS BY VAN OSTAIJEN (IN CHRONOLOGICAL ORDER)

Music-Hall. Antwerpen, 1916.

"Beeldende Kunst. Marten Melsen," *Ons Land,* IV, No. 39 (28 January 1917).

"Schoone Kunsten. Oscar en Floris Jespers I, II," *Ons Land,* IV, No. 43 (February 1917).

"Schoone Kunsten. Oscar en Floris Jespers," *Ons Land,* IV, No. 45 (10 March 1917).

"Schoone Kunsten. Naar aanleiding der tentoonstelling van Paul Joostens," *Ons Land,* IV, No. 47 (24 March 1917).

Het sienjaal. Antwerpen, 1918.

"Kanttekeningen bij diverse onderwerpen," *De Goedendag,* XXIV, Nos. 4–5 (May–June 1918), 47–59.

Bezette Stad. Antwerpen, 1921.

"Boekbesprekingen. Duco Perkens: Het roerend bezit, met tekeningen van Oscar Duboux. Duco Perkens: Kwartier per dag, boekverluchting door Jozef Peeters. Uitg. De Driehoek. Lambrecht Lambrechts: Kleine keuze onuitgegeven gedichten. Henri Bruning: De sirkel. Verzen. Nijmegen in eigen beheer, 1924. Gerard van Duyn: De verlaten stad, met tekeningen door Gerard Rutten. (Amsterdam). Roel Houwink: Novellen. (Zeist)," *Het Overzicht,* Nos. 22–24 (February 1925), 171–175.

Vogelvrij. Grotesken. Antwerpen, 1928.

Gedichten, ed. Gaston Burssens. Antwerpen, 1928.

Intermezzo. Antwerpen, 1929.

Krities proza I, ed. Gaston Burssens. Antwerpen, Utrecht, 1929.

Krities proza II, ed. Gaston Burssens. Antwerpen, Utrecht, 1931.

De bende van de Stronk, ed. Gaston Burssens. Antwerpen, 1932.

Brieven uit Miavoye, ed. Gaston Burssens. Antwerpen, 1932.

Diergaarde voor kinderen van nu, ed. Gaston Burssens. Antwerpen, 1932.

Self-defense, ed. Gaston Burssens. Antwerpen, 1933.

Gedichten, ed. Gaston Burssens. 2d ed. Antwerpen, 1935 (3d ed. 1942).

Verzameld Werk, ed. Gerrit Borgers. 4 vols. Antwerpen, Den Haag, Amsterdam, 1952–1956.

Music-Hall. Een programma vol charlestons, grotesken, polonaises en dressuurnummers, ed. Gerrit Borgers. Den Haag, Antwerpen, 1955 (2d ed. 1957; 3d ed. 1964).

De bende van de stronk. Een romantisch verhaal van roof en liefde gevolgd door

Het bordeel van Ika Loch en De gehouden hotelsleutel, of De kleine domme daad, ed. Gerrit Borgers. Den Haag, Antwerpen, 1957 (2d ed. 1965).

"Portret van een jonge maeceen," ed. Gerrit Borgers. *Maatstaf,* X, No. 7 (October 1962), 431–435.

Verzameld werk. Poëzie 1, ed. Gerrit Borgers. 2d revised ed. Den Haag, Antwerpen, 1963 (3d revised ed. 1965).

Verzameld Werk. Poëzie 2, ed. Gerrit Borgers. 2d revised ed. Den Haag, Antwerpen, 1963 (3d revised ed. 1965).

Verzameld werk. Proza I, ed. Gerrit Borgers. 2d revised ed. Den Haag, Antwerpen, 1966.

De trust der vaderlandsliefde en andere grotesken, ed. Gerrit Borgers. Den Haag, 1966.

Poesie. [flämisch/deutsch] Übertragung und Nachwort von Klaus Reichert. Frankfurt am Main, 1966.

Grotesken, Übertragung von Gerda/Dyserinck-Siecke. Frankfurt am Main, 1967.

Letters

"Een onuitgegeven brief. Paul van Ostaijen tegenover de Vlaamsche Vereniging van Letterkundigen." *De Morgenpost,* July 16, 1932.

"Epistolaire verkenningen. Een briefwisseling tussen Paul van Ostaijen en E. Du Perron uit 1925," ed. Gerrit Borgers. *Maatstaf,* V, No. 10 (January 1958), 641–655.

"Et voila: een inleidend manifest," ed. Gerrit Borgers. *Maatstaf,* II, No. 4 (1952), 253–257.

"Je oordeel is voor mij van waarde. Een briefwisseling tussen Paul van Ostaijen en E. Du Perron uit de jaren 1926–1927," ed. Gerrit Borgers. *Maatstaf,* V, No. 11 (February 1958), 755–772.

"Klare wijn bij een ziekbed. Brieven van E. Du Perron aan Paul van Ostaijen uit het winterhalfjaar 1927–1928," ed. Gerrit Borgers. *Maatstaf,* V, No. 12 (March 1958), 787–801.

"Bij vier brieven van Paul van Ostaijen," ed. Karel Jonckheere. *Nieuw Vlaams Tijdschrift,* No. 10 (1959–1960), 1163–1170.

Floris Jespers, ed. Henri-Floris Jespers. Anvers, 1965.

"Paul van Ostaijens berliniale," ed. Paul de Vree, *De Tafelronde,* XI, No. 1 (January 1966), pp. 2–26.

"Paul van Ostaijen en 'de driehoek'," ed. Paul de Vree. *De Tafelronde* XI, No. 1 (January 1966), pp. 31–37.

SIGNIFICANT STUDIES OF VAN OSTAIJEN'S WORK

Acker, K. van. *Vlaamsche Temperamenten.* Antwerpen, 1944.

Burssens, Gaston. *Paul van Ostaijen, zoals hij was en is.* Antwerpen, 1933.

– *Paul van Ostaijen.* (Monografieën over Vlaamse Letterkunde). Brussel, 1956.

Crub, Geert. "Een posthuum werk van Van Ostaijen," *De Noorderklok,* May 22, 1932.

Gijsen, Marnix. *De literatuur in Zuid-Nederland sedert 1830.* Antwerpen, 1945.

Gilliams, Maurice. *Vita Brevis. Verzamelde Werken.* 4 vols. Antwerpen, 1959.

Gomperts, H. A. *De Geheime Tuin.* Amsterdam, 1963.

Hadermann, Paul. *De kringen naar binnen. De dichterlijke wereld van Paul van Ostaijen.* Antwerpen, 1965.

Kemp, Bernard. *De Vlaamse letteren tussen gisteren en morgen (1930–1960).* Hasselt, 1963.

Minderaa, P. *Opstellen en voordrachten uit mijn hoogleraarstijd (1948–1964).* Zwolle, 1964.

Muls, Josef. *Melancholia.* Antwerpen, 1929.

Passel, Fr. van. *Het tijdschrift RUIMTE (1920–1921) als brandpunt van humanitair expressionisme.* Antwerpen, 1958.

Paul van Ostaijen. Essays by Josef Muls, E. Du Perron, Jan Engelman, Martinus Nijhoff, Maurice Gilliams, Gaston Burssens, J. J. Klant. Antwerpen, Den Haag, Amsterdam, 1952.

Perron, Edgar du. *Verzameld Werk,* ed. E. du Perron-de Roos, F. E. A. Batten and H. A. Gomperts. 7 vols. Amsterdam, 1954–1959.

Rodenko, Paul. "De andere Paul van Ostaijen," *Nieuwe Rotterdamsche Courant,* April 9, 1955.

Roover, Adriaan de. *Paul van Ostaijen.* Brugge, Utrecht, 1963.

Schoonhoven, Etienne. *Paul van Ostaijen. Introduction à sa poétique.* Anvers, 1951.

Stuiveling, Garmt. *Uren zuid: Drie dozijn ontmoetingen over de grens.* Hasselt, 1960.

Tralbaut, Mark Edo. *Van Gogh-reflekties op Van Ostaijen.* Deurne, n.d.

Uyttersprot, Herman. "Kanttekeningen bij Van Ostaijen en het Verzameld Werk," *Spiegel der Letteren,* III, Nos. 3–4 (1959), 225–259.

– *Paul van Ostaijen en zijn proza.* Antwerpen, Rotterdam, 1959.

– *Uit Paul van Ostaijens Lyriek.* Brussel, n.d. [1964].

– "What's in a name. Schmoll en Scheerbart," *De Vlaamse Gids,* XI (1966), 557–567.

Vree, Paul de. "Paul van Ostaijen en de plastische kunsten," *De Tafelronde,* I, No. 7 (July 1953), 365–372.

– "Paul van Ostaijens Berliniale," *De Tafelronde,* XI (January 1966), 2–26.

– and Henri-Floris Jespers, *Paul van Ostaijen.* Brugge, Antwerpen, 1967.

Westerlinck, Albert. *Wandelen al peinzend.* Hasselt, 1965.

NOTES

A LABYRINTH FOR OUR TIMES

[1] G. R. Hocke, *Die Welt als Labyrinth* (Hamburg, 1957), p. 73.

[2] Arthur Clayborough, *The Grotesque in English Literature* (Oxford, 1965), p. 36.

[3] Friedrich Dürrenmatt, *Theater-Schriften und Reden* (Zürich, 1966), p. 128.

[4] John Ruskin, *Modern Painters*, 1st American Ed. (New York, 1865), p. 96. See also "The Grotesque Renaissance," Ruskin's appendix to *The Stones of Venice*, Brantwood Edition, 2 vols. (New York, 1891), II, pp. 187–208. Note that Ruskin's division of the "noble" and the "base" grotesque includes a correlation to the modern grotesque. For Ruskin the "noble" grotesque has beauty, "Nature," and "Mercy." But the "ignoble grotesque," having none of these attributes, corresponds to the modern grotesque in that it "has no pity." Ionesco, speaking of his antitheatre, appears to agree with Ruskin: "Le comique n'offre pas d'issue." Eugène Ionesco, "Expérience du théâtre," *La Nouvelle Revue Française*, VI (February 1958), 260.

[5] "Über Ronald Searle," in *Theater-Schriften*, p. 289. A commentator on modern art indicates how the most ugly aspect of life is acceptable artistically in the form of caricature. "Das hässliche wird selbst von dem langweiligsten Schönheits-Schulmeistern geduldet, wenn es gleichzeitig Komisch wirkt: also ganz besonders im Komischen Genrebild, in der lustigen Bauernszene – in der Karikatur." E. W. Bredt, *Hässliche Kunst?* (München, n.d.), p. 12.

[6] George Santayana, *The Sense of Beauty* (New York, 1896), p. 256.

[7] Wolfgang Kayser, *Das Groteske in Malerei und Dichtung* (Hamburg, 1960); orig. ed. *Das Groteske; seine Gestaltung in Malerei und Dichtung* (Oldenburg, 1957). The American scholar L. B. Jennings is critical of Kayser's work and proceeds to list a number of articles which are unfavorable to Kayser. L. B. Jennings, *The Ludicrous Demon* (Berkeley and Los Angeles, 1963), pp. 157–158.

[8] Jennings, pp. 153–154. Italics added.

[9] Karl Otten, *Expressionismus-grotesk* (Zürich, 1962), pp. 9–10.

[10] Otten, p. 10. Compare the following comment: "Castiglione empfiehlt schon die 'Umkehrung' aller Logik. Er meint, alles werde schöner, 'dicendo ogni cosa al contrario,' wenn man alles auf 'umgekehrte' Weise sage." Hocke, p. 22.

[11] This letter was published in *De Tafelronde*, XI (January 1966), pp. 2–4. Perhaps Van Ostaijen's assimilation of Expressionistic and Dadaistic work during his stay in Berlin explains his anti-naturalistic opinions about literature and art. Before he arrived in Berlin, though already intrigued by the big city, he still could fall victim to a pantheistic adoration of nature, as poems from the volumes of verse from his pre-Berlin years (*Music-Hall*, 1916 and *The Signal* [*Het Sienjaal*], 1918) indicate. But the strong objectivist quality of his major writings must be dated from the Berlin experience.

[12] Otten, p. 13. See also Hocke, especially where he mentions that a simian *leitmotiv* runs through *Manierismus: Die Welt als Labyrinth*, pp. 74–79. Hugo Friedrich postu-

lates an "Ästhetik des Hässlichen" for modern poetry: *Die Struktur der Modernen Lyrik* (Hamburg, 1956), p. 32.

[13] Otten, p. 14.

[14] "Randbemerkungen zur Prosa des Dichters Pasternak," *Slavische Rundschau,* VII, No. 6 (1935), 357–374. This is Jakobson's only detailed formulation of his extremely important theory.

[15] Albert Soergel, *Dichtung und Dichter der Zeit, eine Schilderung der deutschen Literatur der letzten Jahrzehnte. Neue folge. Im Banne des Expressionismus* (Leipzig, 1925), pp. 859–860.

[16] Van Ostaijen writes from Berlin (April 1919): "The greatest German writer is Paul Scheerbart. He writes beautiful hippopotami-asteroids and other novels. Incredibly human and cosmic." Letter published in *De Tafelronde,* XI (January 1966), p. 4. And again in a letter from June 1919: "Scheerbart is wonderful." *De Tafelronde,* XI (January 1966), p. 5. On one occasion Van Ostaijen quotes Scheerbart from his "Nilpferden-roman" (*Verzameld Werk: Proza II,* p. 220). The novel of Scheerbart's he is referring to is *Immer Mutig!,* 2 vols. (Minden in Westfalen, 1902).

[17] Soergel, p. 66. For suggested influences of Meyrink on Van Ostaijen, see H. Uytterspot, *Paul van Ostaijen en zijn proza* (Antwerpen, 1959), pp. 18–19.

[18] Soergel, pp. 72–73.

[19] Kayser, p. 111. Note the following comment by Spitzer about Morgenstern's art: "Der Dichter verhindert die Sprache daran, in ihren Bindungen und Trennungen tot zu verharren, sein 'Spiel' bringt Bewegung in den totruhigen 'Ernst' der Sprache." From "Die groteske Gestaltungs- und Sprachkunst Christian Morgensterns," in Hans Sperber and Leo Spitzer, *Motiv und Wort; Studien zur Literatur-Sprachpsychologie* (Leipzig, 1918), p. 96. One may be reminded here that such was also the avowed intention of Dada. Compare, for example, the poems of Hugo Ball and Tristan Tzara. Hugo Friedrich sees this phenomenon as being axiomatic for modern art *in tota,* especially poetry. "Sofern die moderne Lyrik sich überhaupt noch in ihrem Verhältnis zum Leser definiert, definiert sie sich gerne als Angriff. Der Riss zwischen Autor und Publikum wird durch Schockeffekte offen gehalten. Sie spielen sich ab im abnormen Stil der 'neue Sprache'." Friedrich, *Die Struktur,* p. 115. An example might be the work of the fine contemporary German poet Paul Célan.

[20] For Mynona's optimism see his *Die Bank der Spötter* (München & Leipzig, 1919) and *Der Schöpfer* (München, 1920). It is now a definite fact that Van Ostaijen knew this intellectual Dr. Jekell/Mr. Hyde personally. He became well acquainted with the professor of philosophy (Dr. Salomon Friedlaender) who doubled as the writer of acid grotesques under the name of Mynona, as becomes clear from a letter from Berlin (June 1919): "With Mynona I am now better acquainted. He is a wonderful man. We're organizing a couple of parties shortly." Published in *De Tafelronde,* XI (January 1966), p. 5. Several times Van Ostaijen quotes Mynona in his own work (cf. *Verzameld Werk: Proza* II, pp. 137, 160, 184). It is an intriguing question how much influence the German philosopher/writer had on his young Flemish friend. For example, how much of the discernible parallels with modern philosophical movements (discussed in the final section of this study) are the result of the German writer's influence? Husserl's first published investigations into phenomenology date from 1913. One would assume that a professor of philosophy in Berlin would be at least aware of this new development in his discipline, and might have imparted the knowledge to his Flemish friend who was always notorious for his enormous appetite for new ideas. That Van Ostaijen met Mynona personally is not surprising. Despite his academic profession, Mynona was a well-known figure among Berlin Dadaists at the time. His grotesques were "staple Dada fare," as Hans Richter puts it in his *Dada: art and anti-art* (New York, n.d. [1966]).

[21] Bruce Jay Friedman in his introduction to the anthology *Black Humor* (New York, 1965), p. viii.

²² William Van O'Connor, *The Grotesque: An American Genre and Other Essays* (Carbondale, 1962), p. 3.

²³ Dürrenmatt, p. 194.

²⁴ Jan Kott, *Shakespeare our Contemporary* (Garden City, New York, 1966), p. 132.

²⁵ Hugo Friedrich, *Die Struktur*, p. 143.

²⁶ Johan Huizinga, *Homo Ludens* (Haarlem, 1958).

²⁷ Dürrenmatt, p. 89.

²⁸ Schiller, in *Über naive und sentimentalische Dichtung* (1795), already noted the accent on cerebrality in the comic mode of literature. "Der Tragiker muss sich vor dem ruhigen Räsonnement in acht nehmen und immer das Herz interessieren; der Komiker muss sich vor dem Pathos hüten und immer den Verstand unterhalten." (Reclam edition [Stuttgart, 1963], p. 47) Uytterspot calls Van Ostaijen's grotesques a "verdichtete Logik." H. Uyttersprot, *Paul van Ostaijen en zijn proza*, p. 21.

²⁹ Walter Muschg, "Ernst Barlach als Erzähler," in *Von Trakl zu Brecht* (München, 1961), p. 261.

³⁰ Mark Spilka, *Dickens and Kafka: a mutual interpretation* (London, 1963), p. 71. Kott's interpretation of *King Lear* as a grotesque play, would refute any such "assertive spirit." As he puts it: "The Fool knows that the only true madness is to regard this world as rational." Kott, *Shakespeare*, p. 167.

³¹ Dürrenmatt, p. 136.

³² "The grotesque is the vision of an absurdity, usually of cosmic dimension, which defies all intellectual efforts to clarify and elucidate its possible meaning in terms of human understanding." Karl S. Guthke, *Modern Tragicomedy* (New York, 1966), pp. 73–74.

³³ Dürrenmatt, p. 186.

³⁴ Dürrenmatt, p. 123.

³⁵ G. R. Hocke, *Manierismus*, p. 210.

³⁶ Leslie Fiedler, *No! in Thunder. Essays on Myth and Literature* (Boston, 1960), p. 17.

³⁷ Otten, p. 14.

UNITY OF THEME: A TOPOGRAPHY OF THE GROTESQUE

¹ Garmt Stuiveling, *Uren Zuid* (Hasselt, 1960), pp. 68–70.

² Citations from Van Ostaijen in the text are from the collected works: *Verzameld Werk*, ed. Gerrit Borgers, 4 vols. (Antwerpen, Den Haag, Amsterdam, 1952–1956). This edition has been divided into two sections of "poetry" and "prose" of two volumes each. To maintain such a division would result in confusion, hence for reasons of clarity and common sense, the afore-mentioned edition is referred to as if it were a uniform one by a Roman numeral for each of the four volumes. A second, revised edition of the collected works is being published. But, unfortunately, the last volume is still wanting at the present time. This edition is more inclusive than the former and always prints the first known original of the texts. Between 1963 and 1966, three of the four volumes have been printed. The last, containing all of Van Ostaijen's critical work, promises to print those pieces which in the earlier edition were omitted. Page references to Van Ostaijen's work appear almost always in the text, in order to reduce superfluous footnotes.

³ From a letter to Geo van Tichelen, dated April 1919. This, probably the earliest letter from Van Ostaijen's sojourn in Berlin, has been printed in *De Tafelronde*, XI, no 1 (1966), pp. 2–4.

⁴ Aldous Huxley in his essay on "Breughel" parallels some of Van Ostaijen's interpretations, without presenting Breughel as a painter of the grotesque. Though Huxley

may still call Breughel "the natural historian of the Flemish Folk," a painter of that "peculiarly Flemish scatological waggery," whose art is an "anthropological type of painting," he also senses a reflective side to the Flemish master. Huxley notes that "Breughel's later pictures, painted when he had really mastered the secrets of his art, are not comic at all." The British writer also agrees with Van Ostaijen's view that Breughel's figures are more contour than substance. "All the objects in his pictures (which are composed in a manner that reminds one very much of the Japanese) are paper-thin silhouettes arranged, plane after plane, like the theatrical scenery in the depth of the stage." Huxley merely hints at a grotesque element in his statement that "seen thus, impassively, from the outside, the tragedy does not purge or uplift; it appalls and makes desperate; or it may even inspire a kind of gruesome mirth." Note how similar the last statement is to Van Ostaijen's discussion of Breughel's style. Aldous Huxley, *Collected Essays* (New York, 1958), pp. 135–144.

⁵ Mynona [pseud. Salomon Friedlaender], *Rosa die schöne Schutzmannsfrau* (Leipzig, 1913), p. 19.

⁶ Stuiveling, *Uren Zuid*, pp. 69–70.

⁷ Gerrit Borgers in his introduction to the anthology of grotesques and poems by Van Ostaijen, *Music-Hall* (Den Haag, Antwerpen, 1964), p. 20.

⁸ "The Gang of the Trunk" attracted some attention when it was published posthumously in a collection of grotesques bearing the same title (1932). This particular story dealt satirically with the Belgian Royal Family. A vehement denunciation of Van Ostaijen came from a certain "Rip," who castigated the story as "vieselijk proza, deze smerige smaad tot den Koning en Koningin der Belgen ... walgelijke majesteitsschennis ..." From "Dichterverheerlijking?," *De Nieuwe Gazet*, April 2/3, 1932. A sober reply to this patriotic outburst was supplied by Geert Crub who had understood the main intention of the story – that Van Ostaijen was writing about a mad era and a world out-of-joint. "... uw tijd, uw leiders en afgoden, zijn en hunne ontaarding waar ze het manke, halve, verstompelde tot ideaal verheffen. Het afgeknotte, verminkte wordt toonbeeld ... zijn beledigingen die geen beledigingen meer zijn maar nuchtere vaststellingen van jammerlijke feiten die ook Van Ostaijen walgden." Geert Crub, "Een posthuum werk van Van Ostaijen," *De Noorderklok*, May 22, 1932.

⁹ H. Uyttersprot, *Uit Paul van Ostaijens Lyriek* (Brussel, n.d. [1964], p. 53.

¹⁰ John Ruskin, something of a super-patriot under Queen Victoria, displays a similar intoxication in his lecture on "War" delivered to the Royal Military Academy in 1866. First he asserts that "all pure and noble arts of peace are founded on war; no great art ever yet rose on earth, but among a nation of soldiers." Then he echoes both Van Ostaijen's character, the Peruvian general Gomes, as well as Huizinga's ludic theory when he describes war as a game, a "grand pastime." Ruskin also resembles Van Ostaijen's general when he asserts that war is the expression of total man, man at his supreme height: "the game of war is only that in which the *full personal power of the human creature* [Ruskin's italics] is brought out in management of its weapons." The Englishman also agrees with Ricardo Gomes, Pameelke, and other characters from the grotesque world, that war is necessary as well as inspiring, and that peaceful debates are a stigma on a nation's honor. "I tell you that the principle of non-intervention, as now preached among us, is as selfish and cruel as the worst frenzy of conquest, and differs from it only by being not only malignant, but dastardly." This lecture by Ruskin was reprinted in the American edition of *The Crown of Wild Olive* (New York, 1874), pp. 79–131. How painfully relevant this sentiment still is can be seen in the contemporary satire by an anonymous American, *Report from Iron Mountain on the Possibility and Desirability of Peace* (New York, 1967).

Literary similarities have been suggested. Uyttersprot speaks of an alleged similarity between Van Ostaijen's grotesque and Gustav Meyrink's "Die Erstürmung von Sarajewo." Outside the fact that both tales deal with things military, there is little to substantiate this view. A more plausible case can be made for Paul Scheerbart's tale "Rakkóx der Billionär," first published in Leipzig in 1901. The billionaire orders the director of his "Erfindungsabteilung" to develop a new idea which would revolutionize military science. The director proposes a very elaborate scheme to form an army of animals. The story can be found in a recent anthology of Scheerbart's major works; Paul Scheerbart, *Dichterische Hauptwerke* (Stuttgart, 1962), pp. 229–231. It has become quite clear from recent epistolary evidence that Van Ostaijen knew and admired Scheerbart's work.

[11] H. Uyttersprot spoke of a comparison between Van Ostaijen's "Overtuiging van Notaris Telleke," and Gustav Meyrink's "Der heisse Soldat." A more fitting parallelism seems to be between Meyrink's story and Van Ostaijen's tale "De Cassette." Both tales deal with atrophied credulity which will not allow any explanation other than a traditional one. Cf. Uyttersprot, *Paul van Ostaijen en zijn proza*, p. 18; and Meyrink, *Des deutschen Spietzers Wunderhorn*, II (München, 1922), pp. 124–129.

[12] Christian Morgenstern, *Stufen* (München, 1918), pp. 97, 215.

[13] In French *purée* means most commonly "mashed potatoes." Besides this culinary meaning there is also the expression "être dans la purée," which is perhaps most closely translated by "being in the soup." The Dutch language has completely absorbed the French word with identical meanings. Figurative meanings are: *in de puree* ("smashed to pieces"), with verbs "to smash up something," "to be in a mess," "to be afraid." It is obvious that a word with such widely known negative connotations is hardly the proper surname for a successful businessman.

[14] Cf. the third volume (*Verzameld Werk. Proza* I) of the 2d, rev. ed. of the collected works, pp. 125–127.

[15] The practice of using pseudonyms is perhaps more common in Europe than in the U.S..Dutch literature has a score of writers working under an assumed name: Marnix Gijsen (J. A. Goris), Johan Daisne (Albert Thiery), Ivo Michiels (H. Ceuppens), Lucebert (Lubertus Swaansdijk), J. B. Charles (W. H. Nagel) and E. du Perron who wrote for a time under the name of Duco Perkens, and was a friend of Van Ostaijen. There are many others. In fact, Van Ostaijen himself appears in this tale under a pseudonym. His real last name may be seen as a combination of *os* ("ox") and *taai* ("tough"). In a witty transposition he writes of himself as Paul van Malskoe (III, 379). *Mals* meaning "tender" (meat) and *koe* "cow."

[16] One can find a definite parallel for Van Ostaijen's anti-Freudianism in Mynona's work. One of the German writer's collection of "Grotesken" is called *Das Eisenbahn-glück oder Der Anti-Freud* (Berlin, 1925), and bears the dedication: "Herrn Professor S. Freud in Wien mit dem Herzinnigsten 'Coeo, ergo sum!' gewidmet." The book sets out to prove that the sex-act is purely an accident. It contains one phrase which sums up both Mynona's and Van Ostaijen's position: "das die reductio ad sexum die reductio ad absurdum bedeutet." (p. 34) It contains a story called "Contre Coeur" (pp. 92–96), which bears a definite resemblance to Van Ostaijen's "De verloren huissleutel." Prof. Katz, the hero of "Contre Coeur," is a physician who is deadly afraid of catching syphilis; he suffers, as Mynona puts it, from "Syphilidophobie." The good doctor prescribes himself monastic abstinence. One day a prostitute, Lukrezia, is brought to his clinic with an advanced case of the disease; she is, in fact, "das leibliche Paradigma sämtlicher Luster-krankungen." In a sudden fit of madness, Prof. Katz has intercourse with her. Mynona explains this irrational act by means of a dissertation on the effect on human beings of the law of opposites.

[17] The name Ika Loch can be an anagram for *lochika*, from *logika* meaning "logic." The surname can also have a scurrilous meaning, appropriate to the story and the theme, when one thinks of it as being the German word for a foramen.

[18] Readers might object to the term as being obscure. But see a contemporary dis-

cussion by the British historian Hugh R. Trevor-Roper, "Witches and Witchcraft: An Historical Essay," *Encounter,* XXVIII (May 1967), 3–25.

[19] Uyttersprot in his essay *Paul van Ostaijen en zijn proza* (p. 18) briefly mentions a similarity between "Van een meevallertje dat een malheur was" and Gustav Meyrink't "Bologneser Tränen." The parallel is really quite striking, particularly in Meyrink's description of his heroine Mercedes and Van Ostaijen's Ursula. In the German story, the heroine is called a "Satanistin" and a "Hexe," while one character cries out "welcher Abgrund dämonischer Liebesempfindung lag in diesem Weibe!" Cf. Gustav Meyrink, *Des deutschen Spietzers Wunderhorn,* II, pp. 136–143.

[20] This is true of at least the following tales: "De Bende van de Stronk," "Het Bordeel van Ika Loch," "Werk en Spaar," "Het gevang in de hemel," "Mercurius," "De verloren huissleutel," "Menselijke onvoorzichtigheid," "De kudde van Claire," "De generaal," "De gehouden hotelsleutel," "De man met de zwijnskop," and "Mechtildis." Two stories in this series, incidentally, bear a definite resemblance to two "Grotesken" by Mynona. The latter has a story about a Berlin prostitute entitled "Mechtildis," although the resemblance ends there. There is also a kinship between Van Ostaijen's unfinished piece "De man met de zwijnskop" and Mynona's "Ein Kindes Heldentat." Both German stories can be found in Mynona, *Rosa die schöne Schutzmannsfrau* (Leipzig, 1913), pp. 78–81 and pp. 110–112.

[21] These pages recall a sarcastic remark Van Ostaijen once made in an essay against those who persist in seeing Flemish jollity as an innocent pastime of peasants. "The Kept Hotel Key" may be seen as the fictional answer to his rhetorical question in that essay: "Quand retrouverons-nous Hadewych au bordel?" (IV, 193).

[22] Though very seldom discussed, the curse of mediocrity was emphasized as an insidious evil by Erich Heller. "We have not yet grasped the demonic possibilities of mediocrity. We believe that the only appropriate partner of Mephisto is a genius. It was Karl Kraus who discovered to what satanic heights inferiority may rise. He anticipated Hitler long before anyone knew his name." One should add here Karl Kraus *and* Paul van Ostaijen. Erich Heller, *The Disinherited Mind* (New York, 1959), p. 249.

[23] In a letter to E. du Perron (7 January 1928), published in the collection of letters edited by Gaston Burssens, *Brieven uit Miavoye* (Antwerpen, Amsterdam, 1932), p. 65.

[24] H. A. Gomperts, *De geheime tuin* (Amsterdam, 1963), p. 121. The "publication" referred to are the last two volumes of the collected works: volume III (creative prose) published in 1954, and volume IV (critical prose) published in 1956. Volumes I and II containing the poetry were published in 1952.

[25] In the translation "sexton" stands for *coster.* This is a play on words. Van Ostaijen had a specific critic in mind by the name of Dirk Coster (1887–1956), who was a Dutch critic with humanitarian leanings in literature and strongly pronounced moralistic tone and character. Van Ostaijen was not alone in this battle against constricting forces in the literary and social worlds of Flanders and Holland. He became friends with the Dutch novelist and essayist Edgar du Perron (1899–1940) who, with even greater vehemence, waged a life-long battle against his peers in the Establishment. Du Perron was joined by Menno ter Braak (1902–1940), a Dutch essayist and mordant wit, in forming a militant and polemic periodical and movement known as the *Forum*-group (1932–1935). Dirk Coster was noxious to all three kindred spirits. For readers unfamiliar with Menno ter Braak, see my essay "The Critic and Existence: An Introduction to Menno Ter Braak" in the volume *Criticism. Speculative and Analytical Essays,* ed. L. S. Dembo (Madison, Wisconsin, 1968).

THE STYLE OF THE GROTESQUES: A DESCRIPTION OF
LINGUISTIC SUBVERSION

[1] This essay, "Un debat littéraire," is not included in the collected works, but was published previously in book form. Paul van Ostaijen, *Krities proza* II (Antwerpen, Utrecht, 1931), p. 152.

[2] This theory was primarily developed in an essay on Pasternak: Roman Jakobson, "Randbemerkungen zur Prosa des Dichters Pasternak," *Slavische Rundschau*, VII, No. 6, 357–374. If not otherwise indicated, the quotations from Jakobson are from this essay. See also Roman Jakobson and Morris Halle, *Fundamentals of Language* ('s-Gravenhage, 1956), pp. 76–82.

[3] Ostaijen, *Krities proza* II, p. 149.

[4] Kayser, *Das Groteske*, p. 132.

[5] Albert Gleizes and Jean Metzinger, *Du 'Cubisme'* (Paris, 1912), p. 6.

[6] The quotation is from a catalogue for an exposition of this group's work in Amsterdam's Stedelijk Museum, 6 July to 25 September 1951. *de stijl: cat. 81* (Amsterdam, 1951), pp. 24–25.

[7] Vassily Kandinsky, *Über das Geistige in der Kunst* (München 1912), p. 36.

[8] Paul van Ostaijen, "Lambrecht Lambrechts: kleine keuze onuitgegeven gedichten. Henri Bruning: De sirkel. Verzen. Gerard van Duyn: De verlaten stad. Roel Houwink: Novellen," *Het Overzicht*, Nos. 22–24 (February 1925).

[9] Paul van Ostaijen, "Beeldende Kunst Marten Nelsen," *Ons Land*, IV (28 January 1917). See also his essay "Schoone Kunsten. Oscar en Floris Jespers," *Ons Land*, IV (10 March 1917). In a letter from Berlin to Floris Jespers, Van Ostaijen writes quite seriously about the problematic nature of the caricature, even alluding to what he calls a "classical caricature." This letter is in the possession of Floris Jespers' grandson, Henri-Floris Jespers, who showed it to me and allowed me to quote from it.

[10] Baudelaire in a projected preface to his *Fleurs du Mal;* included in Charles Baudelaire, *Fleurs du Mal,* ed. Antoine Adam (Paris, 1961), p. 249. This is the passage which was singled out by Hugo Friedrich as being especially significant and apocalyptic for modern poetry in *Die Struktur der modernen Lyrik* (Hamburg, 1956), p. 43.

[11] Salomon Friedlaender, *Logik; Die Lehre vom Denken* (Berlin, Leipzig, n.d.), p. 73.

[12] Roger Shattuck, *The Banquet Years* (New York, 1961), pp. 334–335.

[13] Paul Rodenko, "De andere Paul van Ostaijen," *Nieuwe Rotterdamsche Courant,* April 9, 1955.

THE FINAL PHASE

[1] The exception is Herman Uyttersprot's discussion of "The Sirens" in his essay *Uit Paul van Ostaijens lyriek* (Brussel, 1964), pp. 50–61. Cf. also Uyttersprot's article "Kanttekeningen bij Van Ostaijen en het Verzameld Werk," *Spiegel der Letteren*, III, Nos. 3–4, 237; Gerrit Borgers' introduction to the anthology *Music-Hall* (Den Haag, Antwerpen, 1964), p. 20; and Paul Hadermann's study *Paul van Ostaijen* (Antwerpen, 1965), pp. 124–125.

[2] Borgers has a similar interpretation. Cf. his intro. to *Music-Hall*, p. 20.

[3] See Borgers' note in volume III, p. 413.

[4] Hadermann agrees with this bibliographical conjecture on p. 125.

[5] Roman Jakobson and Morris Halle, *Fundamentals of language* ('s-Gravenhage, 1956), pp. 76–78; Roman Jakobson, "A Closing Statement: Linguistics and Poetics," in Thomas A. Sebeok, ed. *Style in Language* (Cambridge, Mass., 1960), p. 370 ff. As in previous sections, the quotations from Jakobson are from his Pasternak essay unless

otherwise indicated: Roman Jakobson, "Randbemerkungen zur Prosa des Dichters Pasternak," *Slavische Rundschau*, VII (1935), 357–374.

[6] Jakobson, *Fundamentals*, p. 78.

[7] Ostaijen, *Krities proza* II, p. 153.

[8] *Krities proza* II, p. 150.

[9] In the following outline of phenomenology and its main figures, I draw chiefly upon the following works: William Barrett and Henry D. Aiken, *Philosophy in the Twentieth Century: An Anthology*, III (New York, 1962), pp. 123–302; Pierre Thévenaz, *What is Phenomenology?*, ed. James M. Edie (Chicago, 1962); I. M. Bochénski, *Contemporary European Philosophy* (Berkeley and Los Angeles, 1966); Herbert Spiegelberg, *The Phenomenological Movement. A Historical Introduction*, 2 vols. (The Hague 1965).

[10] Monroe C. Beardsley, *Aesthetics from Classical Greece to The Present* (New York, 1966), pp. 365–366.

[11] Beardsley, *Aesthetics*, pp. 365–366.

[12] Ostaijen, *Krities proza* II, pp. 152–153.

[13] Barrett, III, p. 131.

[14] Barrett, III, p. 134.

[15] Thévenaz, p. 50.

[16] Thévenaz, pp. 46–47.

[17] Ostaijen, *Krities proza* II, p. 151.

[18] Up to this point, the quotations concerning Heidegger were from Thévenaz, pp. 56–59.

[19] Barrett, III, p. 135.

[20] Martin Heidegger, "The Fundamental Question of Metaphysics," reprinted in Barrett, III, p. 235.

[21] Maurice Merleau-Ponty, *Phénoménologie de la perception* (Paris, 1966), p. 516. Hereafter referred to in the text as PP.

[22] Thévenaz, p. 84.

[23] Thévenaz, p. 88.

[24] Thévenaz, p. 88.

[25] Ostaijen, *Krities proza* II, p. 151.

[26] Gaston Bachelard, *La Terre et les Rêveries du Repos* (Paris, 1963), p. 53.

[27] Ostaijen, *Krities proza* II, p. 149.

[28] Gaston Bachelard, *La Poétique de L'Espace* (Paris, 1964), p. 4.

[29] Bachelard, *L'Espace*, p. 2.

[30] Bachelard, *L'Espace*, p. 15.

[31] Bachelard, *L'Espace*, p. 4.

[32] Bachelard, *L'Espace*, pp. 79–80.

[33] Bachelard, *L'Air et les Songes* (Paris, 1965), p. 10.

[34] Ostaijen, *Krities proza* II, p. 152.

[35] Bachelard, *L'Air et les Songes*, p. 13.

[36] Bachelard, *L'Espace*, p. 87.

[37] Cyrena Norman Pondrom, "Kafka and Phenomenology: Josef K's Search for information," *Wisconsin Studies in Contemporary Literature*, VIII, No. 1 (Winter 1967), p. 79. Cf. "Phénoménologie de Kafka" in B. Groethuysen, *Mythes et Portraits* (Paris, 1947), pp. 145–159.

[38] He suggests parallels between Van Ostaijen's "The Prison in Heaven" and Kafka's "Der Hungerkünstler," between Ostaijen's "The City of Builders" and Kafka's "Das Stadtwappen" and "Beim Bau der chinesischen Mauer"; cf. H. Uyttersprot, *Paul van Ostaijen en zijn proza*, p. 20.

[39] Hadermann, *Paul van Ostaijen*, pp. 124–125 (note 28).

40 The chronology of the first translations of Kafka should apparently be:

Milena Jesenská, "Topič," *Kmen* (Prague), IV, No. 6 (22 April 1920), pp. 61–72.

Paul van Ostaijen, "Tot overwegen voor hereruiters," *Vlaamsche Arbeid*, XV, Nos. 5–6 (May/June 1925), pp. 176–178.

Anon., "La metamorfosis I," *Revista de Occidente* (Madrid), III, xxiv (June 1925), pp. 273–306.

Anon., "La metamorfosis II," *Revista de Occidente*, III, xxv (July 1925), pp. 33–79.

Alexandre Vialatte, "La Métamorphose I," *La Nouvelle Revue Française*, XV, No. 172 (January 1928), pp. 66–84.

Alexandre Vialatte, "La Métamorphose II," *La Nouvelle Revue Française* XV, No. 173 (February 1928), pp. 212–231.

Alexandre Vialatte, "La Métamorphose III," *La Nouvelle Revue Française*, XV, No. 174 (March 1928), pp. 350–371.

Giuseppe Menassé, "Un Fratricidio – Un vecchio foglietto – Davanti alla legge – Il nuovo avvocato," *Il Convegno. Rivista di Letteratura e di Arte* (Milan), IX, No. 8 (25 August 1928), pp. 383–390.

Eugene Jolas, "The Sentence," *transition*, No. 11 (February 1928).

41 Heinz Politzer, *Franz Kafka; Parable and Paradox* (Ithaca, New York, 1962), p. 76.

42 Franz Kafka, *Parables; In German and English* (New York, 1947), pp. 75–77.

43 Herman Uyttersprot, "Kanttekeningen bij Van Ostaijen en het Verzameld Werk," *Spiegel der Letteren*, III, Nos. 3–4, 237.

44 Vassily Kandinsky, *Über das Geistige in der Kunst* (München, 1912), p. 44. Hereafter referred to in the text as UGK.

45 Bachelard, *Terre et Repos*, p. 5.

46 Karl Viëtor, *Goethe: The Thinker* (Cambridge, Mass., 1950), p. 39.

47 UGK, p. 28. Kandinsky himself wrote what might be called prose poems, of which some bear resemblance to Van Ostaijen's work. An example is the following piece entitled "Offen":

> Bald im grünen Gras langsam verschwindend.
> Bald im grauen Kot steckend.
> Bald im weissen Schnee langsam verschwindend.
> Bald im grauen Kot steckend.
> Lagen lange: dicke lange schwarze Rohre.
> Langen Rohre.
> Rohre.
> Rohre.

Vassily Kandinsky, *Klänge* (München, 1913), no pagination.

48 Barrett, III, pp. 156–157.

49 Jakobson in *Style in Language*, ed. Thomas A. Sebeok, p. 371.

50 Jakobson in *Style in Language*, p. 370.

51 One must be careful to assign undue significance to this reference. For one thing, *Monsieur Nicolas* is not a novel but an autobiography – at least for the first 12 of this 16 vols. work. Nicolas was the first name of the author, née Nicolas Edme Retif, better known as Restif de la Bretonne (1734–1806). There is the slight possibility that Van Ostaijen referred to this work because of its subtitle which, in a sense, describes the content of "Nicolas." The full title of the French work is: *Monsieur Nicolas, ou le Coeur-humain dévoilé*, first edition published by the author in 16 vols. in Paris from 1794 to 1797.

52 Thévenaz, p. 58.

53 Thévenaz, pp. 46–47.

54 Bachelard, *L'Espace*, p. 15.